Alexa Hagerty is an anthropologist researching human rights, genocide, and technology. She holds a PhD from Stanford University and is affiliated with the University of Cambridge. Her research has received honours and funding from the National Science Foundation and the Mellon Foundation, among others. She has written for publications including *Los Angeles Review of Books, Wired*, and *Social Anthropology*. Museums such as Palais de Tokyo, Paris; Deutsches Hygiene-Museum, Dresden; and Musée de la main, Lausanne have featured her research, which has also  including *The New York Times, The G*

AlexaHagerty.com

Praise for *Still Life*

'Chilling and vital . . . dictators past and future need to know that literal and symbolic cover-ups will be uncovered . . . you might think that the subject of this sensitive and thought-provoking book is of niche interest but, as Ukraine should remind us, it is still troublingly resonant.'
The Times

'Moving and beautiful, harrowing and horrifying . . . a single sentence can stop you in your tracks . . . stark and upsetting, but also deeply humane and shot through with a hard-won wisdom. You will see forensics in a new light.'
New Scientist

'Absorbing . . . multifaceted and elegiac . . . *Still Life with Bones* captures the ethos that drives the search—often tireless and against the odds—for truth.'
The New York Times

'In this meditative ethnography, a social anthropologist . . . delicately explores the art, the science, and the sacredness of exhumation in the aftermath of genocide. . . . Throughout the book, just as in forensics, 'the ritual and the analytical buzz in electric proximity.'
The New Yorker

'Haunted and fascinating . . . lyrical . . . The stories of these excavators of the past are told compellingly in *Still Life with Bones*.'
The New York Times Book Review

'Powerful and harrowing . . . told with clarity, compassion and utmost respect for those cruelly killed and for those who grieve for them.'
The Irish Times

'*Still Life With Bones* is a stunning book, which forces the reader to ask themselves questions about grief, justice, the cruelty humans are capable of, and what it means to be human in the first place. I learnt so much about the quiet but essential work forensic anthropologists are doing as they slowly and carefully uncover the recent, violent, past in many countries, and bring some closure to relatives still searching for their missing loved ones. Dr Alexa Hagerty's writing is beautiful. The dedication of the people she meets shines through, offering hope that there can be some accountability for the crimes that have taken place, as well as a warning to anyone who might carry them out in the future.'
Sally Hayden, author of *The Fourth Time We Drowned*

'Meticulous, luminous, utterly brilliant. The prose is as delicate and sharp as a ribcage, but the book's beating heart is Alexa Hagerty's wise and compassionate voice, a welcome guide through the atrocities she documents. Equally powerful about the horrors we do one another and the care we are capable of, *Still Life with Bones* is essential reading as a human.'
Alex Marzano-Lesnevich, author of *The Fact of a Body*

'Touching, and achingly honest-a most amazing account of training as a forensic anthropologist. When Hagerty talks about "lives being violently made into bones," I defy you not to be moved. The text is unflinching, but then the crimes and the victims deserve nothing less. I guarantee this will make you think long and hard about cruelty and human rights and the dedication and humanity of the forensic scientist.'
Dame Professor Sue Black, author of *All That Remains*

'*Still Life with Bones* will hold readers rapt. Hagerty takes us deeply inside the experience of an anthropologist learning to dispassionately decode scientific clues while never forgetting that in each bone there is a brutally murdered person who still cries. A startling and profound meditation on death and resilience.'
T. M. Luhrmann, author of *How God Becomes Real*

'In this unforgettable debut, Alexa Hagerty reveals the intimacy and sacredness of forensics, revealing it as a task that, despite its Sisyphean nature, is evermore vital to preservation of memory, story, and ritual-a slow, intricate counterweight to the obliterating power of modern violence. *Still Life with Bones* is at once horrifying and impossibly hopeful.'
Francisco Cantú, New York Times bestselling author of *The Line Becomes a River*

'Haunting . . . will stay with you long after the final word.'
Sunday Post

'She is an exceptional writer, eloquently exploring
both the practicalities and the symbolism of her work,
sidestepping clunky metaphors while finding startling
new ones . . . Philosophical, poetic, never mawkish,
Hagerty's book has the makings of a classic.'
The Times Literary Supplement

STILL LIFE
with BONES

GENOCIDE, FORENSICS AND

THE QUEST FOR JUSTICE

IN LATIN AMERICA

Alexa Hagerty

WILDFIRE

First published in 2023 by
WILDFIRE
an imprint of HEADLINE PUBLISHING GROUP

First published in paperback in 2024 by
WILDFIRE
an imprint of HEADLINE PUBLISHING GROUP

4

Portions of this work were previously published in slightly
different forms.
Portions of the chapter 'A Lovely Grave for
Learning' originally appeared in the *Los Angeles Review of
Books* in 2018.
Portions of the chapter 'The Ghosts of Argentina'
appeared in *Terrain* in 2018. Portions of the chapter 'Seven Griefs'
appeared in *Ethos* in 2022.

Cataloguing in Publication Data is available from the British Library

ISBN 978 1 4722 9579 8

Offset in 8.78/14.52 pt Walbaum 12pt by Jouve (UK), Milton Keynes

Printed and bound in Great Britain by Clays Ltd, Elcograf S.p.A.

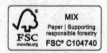

HEADLINE PUBLISHING GROUP
an Hachette UK Company
Carmelite House
50 Victoria Embankment
London
EC4Y 0DZ

www.headline.co.uk
www.hachette.co.uk

For my mother

We have always said that there is the truth under the earth.

—Rosalina Tuyuc

Contents

Following anthropological convention, I have changed the names of all family members and team members, as well as the names of the disappeared. On occasion, I have also altered identifying details to further disguise those individuals. Some people requested that I use their real names, and in those cases, I have done so. Politicians and other public figures appear under their real names.

Articulating Bones

> *There are 206 bones and 32 teeth in*
> *the human body and each has a story*
> *to tell.*
>
> —Dr. Clyde Snow

WHEN I FIRST WASHED BONES in the lab in Guatemala, I was aware that I was touching a part of someone's body. It was disturbing and uncanny. This has faded.

Months later in Argentina, I wash a skull packed with mud. It is hard to remove; I lean over the sink, intent on the work. Suddenly a maggot slithers across my gloved finger. I scream. My lab mates Emilia and Adriana burst out laughing. "Those little gusanos surprise you," says Emilia, who has already pinched the worm between her fingers and tossed it into the trash. "I'll clean the rest," she offers. She would probably like to see if there are more larvae in the cranium. I turn down her offer and go back to work, but the skull seems different now. I feel disgust. The maggot signifies rotting flesh—and it is horrible. I am acutely conscious that I am holding a dead man's head.

Sitting in front of the sinks with Emilia and Adriana, I scrub recognizable bones from spines, legs, and fingers without thinking much of their humanity. I search their surfaces for interesting features, something worthy of closer examination. This detachment isn't just numbness; it is also the product of an increasing fluency "reading" the bones. As a certain form of sensitivity dulls, others grow sharper.

I force myself to keep scooping the mud out of the skull cavity. The revulsion slowly ebbs. I think about how this man saw things through these bony orbits. Just as I am seeing him through holes in bone. With this mandible and maxilla, he drank yerba mate tea, kissed someone, spoke kind words, and said things he regretted. Through these bones he heard a friend call his name and smelled earth after rain. I sponge away traces of dirt. I am careful and thorough, feeling penitent for my disgust and also my detachment.

Forensic exhumation is practiced at the crossroads of two ways of thinking about the dead body: as a scientific object to be analyzed for evidence of crimes against humanity, and as a subject, an individual, someone loved and mourned.

In the lab, forensic anthropologists confront collections of bones and fragments that must be puzzled into a meaningful form. Skeletal remains recovered from mass graves are usually incomplete and often intermingled, meaning that the bones of more than one individual are present. Bones may be broken and eroded. Some are likely to be missing, like the tiny ossicles of the middle ear and the smallest of the twenty-six bones of the feet. Forensic anthropologists "articulate" the skeleton, placing the bones in anatomical order, in the position of someone lying on their back, palms up. Arranging the bones is inevitably an exercise in the partial and incomplete; there are always absences and gaps, elements lost and deteriorated. Anthropologists scrutinize whatever remains, searching for marks of trauma and clues to identity, reading the forensic story the bones tell about a death and a life—their testimony of violence.

Before I set foot in a forensic lab, I associated the term "articulate" with language: the ability to express ideas with clarity or to enunciate words crisply. Bones, like words, can be eloquent. The linguistic root of "articulate" refers to joining together distinct parts, as bones are united by joints and words strung together into sentences. Both words and bones must be arranged in the right order for their meaning to be clear. Bodies and texts are linked, evident in the Latin word "corpus," which means both "body" and a body of literary or artistic work. This root gives us "corpse" and "military corps," with its suggestion of violence, of many bodies and the dead body.

There is a hidden materiality to texts—a word that originally meant "weaving," a connection seen in "texture." Forests haunt writing: The English word for "book" is related to "beech tree" by its Germanic root, and "library" comes from the Latin for "the inner bark of trees." In most Indo-European languages, "writing" comes from carving and cutting. Language carries the memory of words etched into wood tablets, tree trunks, and bones. "Reading bones," as forensic anthropologists do in the lab, is not an analogy so much as a return to the material roots of texts.

The forensic story told in this book explores the matter and meaning of bones: how they are marked by violence and tested in genetic labs. It is also about how bones are always joined to grief, memory, and ritual.

In the late twentieth century, governments in Latin America killed hundreds of thousands of their citizens. Authoritarian leaders directed acts of state terror and genocide against those they labeled as "subversives" and "internal enemies." The catastrophic violence recounted in this book is in the past, but the world is still learning painful lessons about how tyranny leads to atrocity.

The two countries I explore here, Guatemala and Argentina, are different in many ways, but they share a history of "disappearance"—in which people were abducted, tortured, and killed in secret prisons, their bodies discarded in hidden graves. They are also both key sites where forensic human rights practices have been pioneered—developed in the long search for desaparecidos, the disappeared. Latin American forensic teams have led the field, sharing their technical expertise and community-centered approaches with the rest of the world.

In the aftermath of violence, forensic teams exhume mass graves, identify remains, and restore the dead to their families and communities. This is the story of forensic teams working with profound dedication and courage in the face of political impunity and sometimes personal danger. This is the story of families searching for the disappeared and seeking justice—and creating singular forms of mourning and resistance from these twinned pursuits. It is also my story—about how working closely with violence and loss marked me as an anthropologist and person. Like all forensic stories, it is an incomplete inventory, articulated from fragments: fieldwork and archives, formal interviews and late-night conversations, careful field notes and scribbled journal entries; memories I have polished like river stones and memories I can hardly bear to touch. Puzzled together, this book tells the story of the time I spent with families, forensic teams, and the dead.

It is one story among many. Every bone tells a life. Every person lost was a world.

STILL LIFE
WITH BONES

CHAPTER 1

A Lovely Grave for Learning

IT IS SEPTEMBER, and I am standing on a hill in El Quiché, Guatemala, with a pickax in my hand. For the past month, I have been working alongside forensic anthropologists who are recovering the bodies of the victims of one of Latin America's longest, bloodiest armed conflicts. We dig trenches, roughly eight feet long and six feet deep—about the size of a coffin. It is backward grave digging, pulling bodies out of the ground, not putting them in. Plunging the pickax, I imagine hitting a body, and the idea makes me cringe and gives me a visceral reaction of horror. I break my swing and let the pickax land softly on the dirt when I think of this. Before coming here, I had read anthropologist Victoria Sanford's *Buried Secrets: Truth and Human Rights in Guatemala,* an account of her fieldwork in the mid-1990s documenting the aftermath of La Violencia, as the conflict is locally known. At Sanford's first encounter with a mass grave, she repeated to herself: "Don't faint. Don't vomit." I adopt this as my prayer, too. Let us find the bodies, but let me not hit anything— anyone—with a shovel.

Everything begins to look like a body. The white roots of plants and sticks look like bones. Rotted leaves look like fabric; our footprints dried in the mud look like the rubber soles of shoes. Underground, deep down, we find tunnels from moles, colonies of black-winged insects, thick white grubs, and ants. Everything seems like potent proof. And they could be clues. Dead bodies attract these subterranean creatures. There are cycles of life associated with decay. Even after thirty years, when flesh has decomposed, there are still trace nutrients. Like schools of fish in a shipwreck, things take up residence in the armature of bones. As I dig, I think of the lines from *The Tempest*:

> *Full fathom five thy father lies;*
> *Of his bones are coral made;*
> *Those are pearls that were his eyes:*
> *Nothing of him that doth fade,*
> *But doth suffer a sea-change*
> *Into something rich and strange.*

Thousands of men, women, and children are buried in Guatemalan earth, lives violently made into bones, hidden in this strange underground world.

As we dig, forensic team members examine the soil: reddish loam and friable clay. They are looking for evidence that the layers are revuelto, mixed. If the soil has been disturbed, it shows that the area has been previously dug up—potentially a sign of buried bodies. Blended strata mark the earth like a scar. Shoveling is repetitive work, physically exhausting, but not boring. It is electrified by the promise of finding the bodies. But after hours, we still find nothing.

A few times a day, someone unearths pottery shards. We gather around to look at them. One day a farmer brings us a ceramic figure he found while tilling his maize field. The clay head is about the size of a quarter, and the face bears a serious, concerned expression. It looks like something you would see in a museum. It almost certainly should be in a museum. The farmer wants to sell it for 100 USD, but buying it would be illegal. A photographer visiting the site pays him 5 USD to take a picture of it. This haunting little face has been unearthed after being buried perhaps hundreds of years in the sorrowful dirt of Guatemala, where the bones of a decades-old genocide are stacked on top of the bones of five hundred years of colonial conquest. Excavation reveals history as a material presence, the earth as a calendar. We cut through the matted sod of the present, digging through stratified years. Another day, we find part of a clay vessel, its graceful rim nearly intact. Esteban is one of several team members who are classically trained archaeologists and have worked at sites like Tikal and Cotzumalhuapa. He says it is prehispánico, dating it to before the Spanish invaded, greedy for gold, sugar, and slaves. Before what Maya accounts call the arrival of the "force of great suffering" and the beginning of "misery and affliction." Esteban throws the fragment back into the pit, like catch-and-release fishing. It is illegal to take any of the shards. Anyway, they aren't what we are here for.

. . .

THE MASS GRAVES we are searching for are the grim legacy of the armed conflict in Guatemala from 1960 to 1996. I am training with one of the world's top forensic teams, the Forensic Anthropology Foundation of Guatemala, or the Fundación de Antropología Forense de Guatemala, known by its acronym, FAFG. I'm learning how to exhume and identify the dead. Every morning we make the forty-minute drive from the cement-block rooms we're renting in a bigger town through the mountainous province of El Quiché. Villages dot the countryside with clusters of cement schools and houses and stores painted with Coca-Cola signs. Most towns have two or three Evangelical churches, eye-catching because they are the only freshly painted buildings. Mostly we drive past milpa, steep hillsides planted with corn.

We pull over on a deeply rutted dirt road. Esteban hands us pickaxes and shovels from the back of the pickup truck. It has been raining, and the path through the woods is slick. We swing the tools into the muddy ground to anchor our steps, trudging through a tunnel of trees. After a ten-minute walk, the path opens into a field. It's an ordinary field, a rolling meadow ringed by trees. The sky has cleared. With the sun shining, it looks like a good place for a picnic.

It takes a moment to notice the holes in the ground, dozens of short trenches. These are exploratory excavations, abandoned when they yielded no bodies. The holes are half filled with rainwater and trash now. So far, the team has found about twenty bodies in small graves of two or three people, but this is just the beginning. Members of the forensic team guess there are two hundred bodies here under the earth. Maybe more. Mass graves riddle Guatemala. Most are still waiting to be exhumed. Many will never be found.

In the cool morning, we work above the field on a ridge that drops into thick woods. From the excavation site, you can hear but not see a river running nearby. As the crow flies, we are not that far from the nearest town. Across the valley, you can just make out the cemetery with its brightly painted gravestones and its wall of nichos, where the dead rest aboveground in something like a mortuary apartment block. Sometimes strains of music from the local church float to us. It is easy to forget that we are so close to the village. It feels isolated.

In the 1980s, this was the site of Xolosinay, an army garrison long since abandoned. Soldiers detained residents of surrounding villages in the camp. The families of those who were taken here never saw them again. No one knows how many people were killed and buried here. One man managed to escape. The soldiers had ordered the prisoners to dig a trench, then lined them up in front of it and shot them one by one. During the executions, the lone survivor managed to dive into the underbrush. A soldier fired at him, hitting him in the arm, but he fled into the deep woods. He spent years on the run in the mountains.

In the three decades since soldiers held the man prisoner, the site has changed. The soldiers are gone. The tents and paths have disappeared. The trees have grown. But he remembers where he stood in front of the pit of bodies—on the crest of the hill where we are digging.

• • •

AS PART OF the peace process begun in 1996, the United Nations–sponsored Commission for Historical Clarification quantified the staggering toll of the violence in Guatemala. In a country of eight million people, there were 200,000 dead. An estimated 45,000 people had been disappeared. More than a million people suffered forced displacement. There were 626 massacres and 430 villages razed. The truth commission determined the Guatemalan state to be responsible for 93 percent of the documented abuses. More than 80 percent of the victims of the armed conflict were Maya. The commission declared that the state had committed genocide.

The numbers reported by the truth commission are shocking, but they do not capture the cruelty of La Violencia. People told me stories of babies beaten against walls, pregnant women eviscerated, men burned alive, girls raped in front of their families, boys decapitated, people hacked to death with machetes. These gruesome testimonials have been confirmed by truth commission investigations, chronicled by human rights groups, and documented by forensic evidence.

• • •

THE ENORMOUS SCALE of violence in Guatemala leaves forensic teams confronting a daunting task. "Even if 30 forensic teams worked for 30 years, that still wouldn't be enough resources or time to exhume all the mass graves in Guatemala," said Fernando Moscoso, one of the founders of the Guatemalan team. There are about eight FAFG members at the site in Xolosinay at any one time. It is a rotating cast, with people coming and going, leaving to work at other exhumation sites, or returning to the lab in Guatemala City. Although formal systems of training and accreditation are increasing, many forensic anthropologists in Latin America learn their skills in long apprenticeships. Students from a range of disciplines, such as archaeology and biological anthropology, study with teams. You can tell the new archaeologists by the way they dig. They are slow and precise. They excavate layer by layer, attentive to subtle changes in the soil. "It won't last; it takes too damn long," jokes a more experienced team member as we watch a young archaeologist carve a precise corner angle in a deep excavation. "Why don't you add a window and some stairs?" someone yells. They are joking, but there's a hint of irritation. Funding is tight; time is precious. Working fast is imperative to find more bodies.

The FAFG, like most forensic teams, runs on a shoestring budget. They entrepreneurially use their state-of-the-art DNA lab to offer other services, including paternity testing. I am here as part of a field school, hands-on training in forensic anthropology for graduate students. Field schools are an important part of forensic education and also afford forensic teams a much-needed source of extra income. There are three students in our training course, all from different universities in the United States: Nicole, a biological anthropologist; Stephanie, a forensic anthropologist; and me, a social anthropologist. Most field schools are considerably larger. Students from North America and Europe flock to Guatemala. The FAFG is among the world's most respected and accomplished forensic teams, so it is a chance to study with the best of the best. But there's another, more disturbing reason. In Guatemala, forensic students from Europe and North America can see more bodies in a few weeks than in a year back home. Guatemala has so many dead.

In addition to the two hundred thousand people killed during the armed conflict, there are new dead bodies every day. Guatemala City is one of the most violent cities in the world. The 1996 peace accords did not bring peace. Between 2000 and 2006, violence rapidly escalated, with homicide rates nearly doubling and 93 percent of murders left unsolved, leading a UN report to call Guatemala "a good place to commit a murder." A *New Yorker* article on crime and impunity in the country reported, "In 2009, fewer civilians were reported killed in the war zone of Iraq than were shot, stabbed, or beaten to death in Guatemala." Peacetime homicide rates rival death tolls during the armed conflict, leaving questions about what "postwar" really meant. It wasn't just that violence continued unabated; it was also that many of the same actors carried out the killings. State death squads morphed into criminal cartels.

The violence that hangs over Guatemala City is nearly palpable. Small shops do business through secured doors, passing sodas and cigarettes through bars to customers. On a late-night return from a rural exhumation site, we drive on the main artery into Guatemala City. A body lies sprawled across the center lane of the highway. We slowly pass the dead man, lying in a halo of blood. A gang execution, everyone agrees.

A few weeks after I left Guatemala, I got an email informing me that a team member, a soft-spoken man I crossed paths with at the lab, had been killed. He was stabbed seventeen times, apparently for the money in his wallet and his ten-year-old car. It happened near a fancy mall where we once went for lunch, eating sandwiches on the steps of a new faux-Tuscan shopping emporium. The mall is part of a gated development that promises comfort and safety. The security guards carry concealed weapons, and the cheapest condos sell for seventy times the average Guatemalan's annual salary. Residents say that it gives them a chance to escape the city's violence. The architect puts it more bluntly, saying it "sells an illusion that everything is okay."

There are no illusions at the Guatemala City morgue, which does not have refrigeration and overflows with the dead. There is literally no more room in the municipal cemeteries, where workers aggressively disinter corpses to make space for the newly dead.

. . .

AT THE FIELD school, I quickly learn a new vocabulary of the dead: skeletonized bodies, fleshed bodies, mummified bodies, saponified bodies. It's the saponified bodies that worry me the most. I haven't seen one, but others have, and they describe them in clinical yet lurid detail. Saponification is a form of decomposition in which fat transforms into a rancid, foul-smelling material, technically known as adipocere but also called "grave wax."

I desperately hope that we don't encounter saponified bodies. Sanford's prayer runs through my mind: "Let me not faint or vomit" . . . or cry. I am afraid I will be overwhelmed by horror, disgust, or sadness. If I show my emotions, I'll be marked as weak. I'm the only social anthropologist in the group. My subdiscipline seems a lot less tough than forensics or even archaeology. They excavate earth and analyze bones. We listen to people's stories. Maxi, who leads the field school, jokes, "Why don't you stay here, and we'll teach you to be a real anthropologist?"

. . .

AT THE FAFG lab in Guatemala City, forensic anthropologists carefully piece together exhumed remains, beginning the painstaking identification process. The first skeleton I work with is a "teaching skeleton," a donated or unclaimed body used for forensic training. He is referred to as "the mummy" because his body was found mummified in the municipal dump. His desiccated flesh has been long since stripped away. Many labs have a machine for this purpose, which students jokingly call the "stew pot," but it can also be achieved with scalpels or beetles. When I encounter the mummy, he is a skeleton. A chunk is missing from his spine, a square cut from the bone. I think it must be a mortal wound, but the others laugh and say it's from an operation for a herniated disk. How in one life does a man go from being wheeled through a hospital for back surgery to being left dead at the city dump? No one knows his story.

. . .

BONES ARE SMOOTH and rough; they slide against each other and hang together like a medieval machine. You remember them by saying that this one looks like the Indian subcontinent; this one looks like the head of a bull. Each vertebra has its clues. Ribs fit together in a nested arc. They are jigsaw pieces. Puzzling out the complete skeleton is absorbing and satisfying.

One morning in the lab, a small piece of skin is being passed around to be analyzed and discussed. It is handed from person to person. I see it coming toward me, and I feel sick. I don't want to touch it, but I cannot excuse myself without being obvious. When it arrives, it seems like a piece of tree bark. I can't connect the stiff brown flake to anything human. The bodies are changeable. They flicker in and out of personhood.

A few days later, we are learning about teeth. In determining age, dentition offers essential clues. We study a skull that can be "aged" with precision because the secondary (adult) teeth are visible growing through the jawbone, about to push through. The juvenile teeth are loose. Our instructor removes them, and we take turns holding them in our palms, where they rattle like dice. We examine their shapes: canine, incisor, bicuspid, molar. When we think we know where they go, we position them into sockets in the mandible and maxilla. In the right location, they slip into place, a perfect fit. All at once, she appears, the child whose skull I am holding. She materializes so vividly that it verges on hallucination. She is a girl of five or six, with big brown eyes and bed-head. Then she's gone. Then I touch her teeth like dice again.

My fear of crying begins to be replaced by a new fear. That I won't cry, that I won't feel anything. Is it worse when the child appears or when she does not?

I spend the rest of the afternoon cleaning bones with a tooth-brush and a pan of water. Massive, solid femurs. Tissue-paper bones in the nasal passage. Some bones are porous and fragile; in the water, they take on a soft, fleshy consistency. Touching bones is uncanny and sad. But sometimes it is also like washing mud off sticks.

． ． ．

AT THE EXHUMATION site in El Quiché, families arrive in waves throughout the day, standing and watching above the pits where we are working. Men from the community do most of the digging, which is all by hand. To use machines like backhoes would damage the remains and destroy evidence. Members of the forensic team direct the excavation, indicating where to shovel and when to give up and fill the holes back in.

I often dig with Don Jaime, who is from the local community. The team has hired him to help with the excavation. He is forty years old, with an open face and a gold tooth. He asks me where I'm from.

"California."

"Me too; I lived in the Central Valley for seven years!"

Don Jaime picked lettuce and strawberries in one of the most productive agricultural regions in the United States. California grows more than half the country's fruit and vegetables, and 88 percent of the state's farmworkers were born outside the United States. Don Jaime came back to Guatemala because his wife and son live here. While we work, he likes to practice his English. We exchange words in English, Spanish, and Ixil, one of

Guatemala's twenty-two Mayan languages: "Shovel." "Mud." "Bucket." A vocabulary of the things at hand. We dig together, but at some point, it becomes apparent that he's humoring me. He encourages me to take breaks and drink water, and when I come back, he has dug alone in ten minutes what it took us an hour to dig together. When I point this out, he laughs, "Well, you're not used to it." Stanford University, where I am a PhD student, is about a four-hour drive from the fields where Don Jaime worked.

Don Jaime wants to go back to California. When? Soon. "You can't make any money here." The journey is difficult, but many people try. As James Verini reports in *The New York Times Magazine:* "Guatemalans had been migrating to the United States for decades, but mass migration began in earnest in the 1980s, when the civil war entered a genocidal phase." Crossing the border can be deadly. To discourage migration, the U.S. government secured the parts of the border with Mexico that are easier to enter, like San Diego, which has routed migrants to more dangerous areas like the Sonoran Desert. This did not diminish crossings, but it dramatically increased deaths. Anthropologist Jason De León calls this federal policy "a killing machine," and human rights advocates have declared a "mass disaster" at the border. Don Jaime worries about going to California and worries about staying in Guatemala. His teenage son needs his dad. But the family struggles without the money Don Jaime makes in the United States. Digging for the team is better than most local jobs, but it isn't steady work—they don't excavate all the time. It doesn't matter, Don Jaime tells me, he'd do it for free. His brother disappeared during the armed conflict. He was last seen entering Xolosinay.

Don Jaime tells me his brother's last words when soldiers came to take him away: "They can take my body, but they cannot take my soul."

· · ·

THE VERY LOGIC of disappearance implies that bodies are difficult to recover. In Guatemala, people were buried in unmarked graves. In Argentina, people were thrown from planes into the ocean. In Mexico, bodies are burned with tires. There are many cruel strategies to hide and destroy bodies. The whole point is to make the recovery and identification of bodies difficult, if not impossible. So it is not surprising that even the most rigorous and well-funded forensic exhumation projects tend to have modest success. Typically, teams recover a relatively small number of the missing and the process is slow. In Guatemala, the FAFG has identified 3,781 people in nearly thirty years of work. In Argentina, it has taken almost forty years to recover about 1,400 sets of remains.

Given the difficulty of the task, what is remarkable is the monumental effort applied to the attempt. Observing teams at work, I am struck by the almost superhuman effort that recovering and identifying bodies entails. One night in El Quiché, at the only bar in the little town we're staying in, between jokes and forensic horror stories, I ask Maxi and José, who have both worked with the team for a long time, how many hours it takes to identify a single body. They scribble on napkins, but the hours are almost incalculable. Even if you don't include the time spent searching for the precise location of the graves. Even if you forget about the days Don Jaime and the other men spend digging, the hours the drivers spend transporting the team to the site, the time the women in the community spend cooking everyone lunch every day. Even if you leave aside the trips on barely passable dirt roads to find families to record oral histories and gather DNA samples. Even if you disregard years of legal battles, red tape, and fundraising. If you center your calculations solely on the direct effort to recover bodies, the total hours are staggering.

There is the careful cleaning in place of the remains at the field site and the documentation, measurement, and photography. Then there is the meticulous process of removal when the bodies are sorted into labeled bags and boxes. At the lab, there is more cleaning and the extraction of a piece of bone or tooth for DNA sampling. Finally, the remains are pieced together to discern clues to identity and cause of death.

When put on the spot, Maxi and José hazard a guess that each body requires about a month of effort to exhume and analyze. At that rate, it would take nearly four thousand years of human effort to identify all the disappeared in Guatemala. Seen like this, exhumation is an epic undertaking. It is a quixotic task carried out with scientific precision. Of course, these calculations are only a sort of game—our scribbled napkins end up under bottles of Gallo beer—but they point out the near impossibility of the project. They make it clear that many of those most closely affected by disappearance—parents, partners, even children—will not live long enough to see the return of their loved ones' bodies. There is urgency to the work. Forensic teams are racing against the clock to find and return the missing while there are still living mourners to grieve and bury them.

. . .

ONE MORNING I ask Don Jaime if he would tell me the story of what happened to his family during the conflict. Only if he wants to, I add. I haven't asked anyone for an interview yet. As a social anthropologist, I'm supposed to be interviewing people, but I've been hesitant. It feels like prying into pain. "Yes," he says right away, "I want to."

After lunch, Don Jaime appears in a clean shirt with his hair combed back. Things quickly take shape: People gather, and a photographer visiting the project consults with Don Jaime and sets up a tripod. Someone spreads one of the plastic tarps used to cover graves on the ground like a rug and positions a stump for Don Jaime to sit on, adding to a sense of ceremony. What I had imagined as a private interview has turned into a testimonio, an event with a long history in Latin America, a form of public witnessing about experiences of violence and oppression that sets the story straight.

By the time we are ready to start, about twenty people have crowded around, mostly women from the community, but also people from the team. I am sitting on the tarp in front of Don Jaime, who sits on the stump. A translator who works at the site pulls close. We confer. Don Jaime says he will speak Spanish and the translator will relay the testimonio in Ixil. I set my audio recorder between us and tell Don Jaime that I won't use his real name. Using pseudonyms is standard anthropological practice and all the more necessary in Guatemala, where the legacy of impunity means that perpetrators and victims continue to live side by side, and speaking up about the crimes of the past can have dangerous repercussions in the present.

Exhumations can be political flashpoints. For example, on June 14, 2003, the community of Rabinal gathered to rebury the remains of seventy people exhumed from a mass grave. The area around the Achí Maya village was the site of more than twenty documented massacres, the majority carried out during the two years General Efraín Ríos Montt held power, from 1982 to 1983. People converged in the center of town carrying coffins, but then trucks and helicopters arrived. Soon Ríos Montt himself stepped into the main square, flanked by supporters. He claimed to be making a campaign stop in his bid to run in the presidential election, but local families interpreted his arrival as an attempt to intimidate and silence them.

"Use my real name," Don Jaime says, not so much to me but to the people gathered around. "I am not afraid; I will tell my story." Then he turns to me and says in English, "Well, use my first name." This is the last question I ask because Don Jaime, which is not his real name, straightens his back and begins to speak. There is no pause, no time for questions; it is his story, his testimonio.

"What I am going to say is real, it is the truth, and I saw it with my own eyes when I was twelve years old. I was very young, but I remember very well." Don Jaime's family had decided to move from their village to a more remote area. His parents were worried about the steady influx of the military, especially the Kaibiles, an army special forces unit notorious for their brutality.

Don Jaime's father woke up early one Monday morning to look at a piece of land. Don Jaime insisted on accompanying him, and they began hiking into the mountains. Thirty minutes outside their village, at about 5:30 A.M., they heard two explosions. Don Jaime recognized the sound as grenades, but his father tried to convince him it was only fireworks from a nearby village celebrating a fair day. They took a few more steps along the path before hearing the unmistakable sound of sustained gunfire. From their vantage point, they could see thick smoke rising from their village and knew that the soldiers had begun to burn houses and fields, a common scorched-earth tactic.

Don Jaime and his father waited, thinking that people from the village would escape along the path they were on. People passed them, but Don Jaime's mother and his brothers and sisters were not among them. "I felt a knot in my throat. I felt something so heavy in my heart. I knew then that my mother must have died." Eventually, they left the path to hide in the woods, afraid of being discovered by the soldiers.

The next day at dawn, Don Jaime and his father made their way back to their village. They found Don Jaime's mother lying dead in their house. "She was covered in blood, and she was totally exposed to the morning cold. My baby brother was still on her back, and he'd been shot. They had shot her in the stomach and the back, and the bullets had come out through her heart." At the neighbor's house, they found a scene of intense carnage. One of the daughters of the family, a girl about Don Jaime's age, had been decapitated. "We thought maybe dogs had eaten her, but it wasn't dogs. It was grenades that did that to her, cut off her head." At another house, they found a woman lying faceup, holding her eight-month-old baby. "They killed them both with one bullet," says Don Jaime. "This is the truth I'm telling you."

When Don Jaime finishes his testimonio, we all sit in silence, except for the thud of shovels and pickaxes behind us and the sound of the river we cannot see. An older woman named Doña María, who comes to the site most days, has been listening and says that she would like to give her testimonio, too. Like most women from the community who visit the site, she is wearing traje, traditional clothing that varies by region but usually consists of an embroidered top, known as a huipil, and a corte, a skirt made from a large piece of folded fabric. Her daughter helps her to the stump, gingerly crossing the slippery plastic tarp. Doña María is not fluent in Spanish. The translator moves close. Doña María leans near the audio recorder and states her name, first and last. Then she says, in Spanish, to make sure everyone understands: Fue en el mes de octubre, tres de octubre, en día sábado—It was in the month of October, the third of October, a Saturday—before switching to Ixil to give her testimonio about the murder of her husband and two sons.

For the rest of the afternoon, people take turns telling their stories, seven in all, relating experiences of profound violence and loss, testifying to the wounds of La Violencia.

．．．

AFTER FOUR DAYS of digging at the site, we have found nothing. Esteban and other senior team members decide that we will be allowed to exhume remains that have already been located but not yet recovered. We are students, we need bodies to learn, and we won't be in the field forever. I hear rumors that the team has not yet exhumed the bodies because journalists from *The New York Times* are coming to visit the site, and they want to be sure there is something for them to see. Nicole, Stephanie, and I whisper among ourselves: Is it theatrics to "perform" an exhumation for journalists? Is it fair to delay an exhumation since families are waiting for the return of their loved ones? More experienced members of the team accept the situation with a pragmatic shrug. The journalists won't wait days or weeks for the team to find bodies. A newspaper article will raise awareness, help with fundraising, and tell the families' stories. As for the delay, the process is long, and a few weeks won't matter much. Even after the team finds remains, it can take months and sometimes years to clear all the legal and bureaucratic hurdles for their return to families and communities.

We start digging in the softer dirt of a partially excavated area. Our shovels hit plastic soda bottles. This confuses me until I realize that the team used the bottles to mark the depth where they found the remains and then covered everything back over with earth for protection. We shift from digging dirt as fast as we can to working slowly, with care. Setting our shovels aside, we kneel and remove the soil with gardening spades and our hands. Vicente, an experienced team member who has come over to guide us, exposes the edge of a bone and some blue fabric. Even though I know that bodies are buried here, it doesn't seem real. I feel shaky. *Don't faint or vomit.*

People, women and children mostly, gather around to watch us work. We fill plastic colanders with dirt and pass them to José, who inspects them, running his fingers through the dirt, looking for teeth and the small bones of the hands and feet. Our tools get even smaller: toothbrushes, chopsticks, bamboo skewers, paintbrushes, and our fingertips. José directs us—use a brush now, stop there, leave some earth in place for support. Within an hour, the distinct forms of bodies are visible. Two bodies are directly on top of each other, and one is slightly to the side. All are skeletonized, meaning the flesh has decomposed and only bone is left.

I am assigned the job of cleaning the legs of the uppermost body. Based on a preliminary examination of the jaw and skull shape, Nicole says the body appears to be male. José nods. I can't tell from the skeleton, but tattered men's work clothes cover the bones. After about an hour, we change roles. Exhumation requires holding yourself in uncomfortable positions, and it is a relief to assume a new posture. I now work on the top part of the body. As I sweep away the dirt with a soft brush, I see that what initially appeared to be a single skull is two crania, one on top of the other. The lower one seems intact, at least so far, but the upper one is shattered. There is a bullet casing in the soil nearby. I slowly uncover several inches of the lower skull and then work along his shoulder and arm. I carefully dislodge the dirt with the stem of a toothbrush and brush it away with the bristles, slowly revealing a blue-and-red plaid shirt. The colors are bright, the fabric intact, and the buttons still tightly stitched in place. I wonder about the people standing above the grave watching; could someone recognize the shirt?

The first hours of work have been done in near silence, but now the people observing are chatting and talking on their phones. Sounds from the nearby town float up through the valley: off-key heartfelt church singing and the mechanical oompah-pah music of an ice cream truck. There is no funerary feeling, no sense that there should be silence. But there is something—an intensity, a contained outrage. Vicente says with fury that there are at least five bodies here. Five.

There is a sense of excitement, too. It grows as we expose the bodies. Everyone working at the site comes over. Are there signs of trauma? Yes. Two of the bodies have shoes. Look carefully to see the position of the hands. That can tell you a lot: Are they bound, at their sides, covering their faces? The most exposed body has a rope ligature tying his wrists behind his back. Esteban remarks to Maxi that it is una bonita fosa para aprender—a lovely grave for learning.

Using a chopstick to loosen the earth, I follow the outline of the leg, sweeping the dirt into a plastic dustpan and then dumping it into the colander. José instructs me to work from the knee in both directions. Through the fabric of the pants, the shinbone is familiar; it's the same feeling as rubbing my leg, only the ridge of bone is sharper. But if my hand slips around the side of the leg, where his calf should be, there is nothing. I put all my focus on the tip of the chopstick and the bristles of the paintbrush. When I reach the feet, José tells me to go slow and take care: The bones are small, easily disturbed, and easy to miss or throw away. Fortunately, the body is wearing boots. Socks and shoes are "lucky" to find because they trap the small bones and hold them together in tidy packets that can be unwrapped and pieced together in the lab. The boots are perfectly preserved. I scrape mud from the treads, noticing how the heel is worn down. I look up from the grave. Don Jaime and other men from the community are standing by the edge watching, taking a break from shoveling. They are all wearing the same rubber boots as the dead man.

CHAPTER 2

Forensic Lamentations

T HE BUREAUCRAT at the Public Ministry directs his assistant to empty two boxes of evidence so that he can examine the contents. From the cardboard boxes labeled with case numbers, she impassively pulls dirt-stained shirts, faded skirts, and stiff blankets, everything that was found with the bodies. She arranges the fabric, fragile and musty from its long burial, on the floor between the desks and filing cabinets. The bureaucrat nudges a still-intact plastic sandal with his polished shoe and says: "There are too many clothes for two people." He shakes his head, suspicious.

I have been at the Ministry all morning with Alvaro, one of the senior members of the forensic team, and Zulma, a social worker and activist in a Maya human rights organization. We came to pick up the boxes, and what was supposed to be a fifteen-minute errand has turned into an hours-long wrangle with red tape. We follow the bureaucrat back to his office. He is young, barely thirty, but carries himself with middle-aged authority and paunch. He is taller and paler than most people in town. He seems new to the job, and I wonder if he has recently been posted from the capital. While he makes another phone call to Guatemala City, we wait, sitting in a line of chairs across from his desk like naughty students in the principal's office. The bureaucrat talks on the phone, reading off the case numbers to someone on the other end of the line.

Through the glass office door, I watch office staff step over the fabric lying on the ground. The mother and son whose clothes are spread on the floor and whose bones sealed in the boxes were exhumed four years ago. Since then, the case has been winding its way through scientific and legal pathways. Everything has led to this day: the weeks of shoveling, DNA tests from cheek swabs and bone samples, oral histories and testimonios, court orders and case numbers—years of labor culminating in this moment when the family can finally reclaim and bury the bodies— "inhumation," in forensic terms. All that stands in the way of a dignified funeral now is this small-town bureaucrat.

• • •

AS PART OF the peace process that began in 1996, truth commissions and human rights groups urged the Guatemalan government to find and identify the victims of the genocide. The government never did. It has always been the Guatemalan forensic team FAFG, not the government, leading the search for those killed in La Violencia.

In 1998, the Recovery of Historical Memory project, led by Bishop Juan José Gerardi Conedera and sponsored by the Catholic Church, released its investigation of La Violencia. Titled *Guatemala: Nunca Más (Guatemala: Never Again)*, the explosive 1,400-page report was based on more than 6,500 witness testimonies and documented more than 55,000 victims. It also named perpetrators. State-sponsored exhumations were among its recommendations: "Families have the right to exhume their dead and this right should be officially guaranteed, given that the army was directly responsible for the vast majority of clandestine burials." In his public presentation of the report, Bishop Gerardi told the audience packed into the Metropolitan Cathedral, "Learning the truth is painful, but it is undoubtedly a highly healthy and liberating act." Two days after *Guatemala: Nunca Más* was published, the military assassinated Bishop Gerardi.

The government was still in the business of making dead bodies, not finding them—and making an example of anyone who tried to bring the crimes of the genocide to light.

Members of the Guatemalan forensic team have repeatedly received death threats, one of which read simply: "Death to the anthropologists." Since its founding in 1992, the nongovernmental organization has been supported by international human rights groups and grants from foundations. Local communities trust the FAFG's independence. Over the years, the team has built good relationships with government bodies such as the Human Rights Unit of the Public Prosecutor's Office.

. . .

THE BUREAUCRAT HANGS up the phone and flips through the stack of papers. Finally, he says, "No, it's impossible. There's a mistake in the paperwork." Alvaro says, "The family is here. They were told to come today." He speaks calmly, even though I know he must be frustrated. The bureaucrat leans back in his chair and tells Alvaro to bring in the family; he wants to ask them some questions. In the hall, Alvaro and Zulma exchange a look that I interpret as *Here we go*.

"Why are there so many clothes?" the bureaucrat demands. Manuel, a stocky and serious man of about forty, stands in front of his mother's clothes and the blankets used to wrap his little brother's body and tries to explain that in the Maya Cosmovision, the dead need their everyday things in the afterlife.

In 1982, Manuel's family fled their village. Soldiers shot and killed Doña Asunción and her six-year-old son, Oscar, as they ran across an open field toward the cover of forest. Manuel, twelve at the time, made it to the trees and survived.

At great risk, Manuel, his father, and other men from his village snuck back to the field at night to bury his mother and brother where they'd been cut down. During the violence, soldiers often forbade people from burying the dead, threatening that anyone touching the bodies would be killed, too. Bodies were left for days in streets and fields, to fester and be eaten by dogs. It was dangerous to return to bury Doña Asunción and Oscar; the area was crawling with soldiers. But the men and boys dug a grave and buried mother and son with quick prayers and the provisions they could manage as funeral custom demanded. The blankets, clothes, and other supplies they gave were of desperate use to the living. People hiding in the mountains died from cold and hunger. But leaving the dead exposed was unbearable. Manuel and the other men risked death to bury the bodies with dignity.

The objects on the floor in front of us, the stiff blankets, the tin cups, and the cinta that Doña Asunción once wore wrapped around her head, its colors still bright even after thirty years underground, are evidence of the profound importance of caring for the dead. "It's the old-fashioned way," Manuel tells the bureaucrat through his daughter, who acts as his interpreter. Manuel is deaf. His daughter translates between sign language and Ixil for the family and Spanish for the bureaucrat.

"He's deaf?" The bureaucrat directs the question to Alvaro, pointing toward Manuel. "Is he literate?" asks the bureaucrat. A flurry of signs passes between Manuel and his daughter. Her father doesn't know how to read, she says. "In that case, he is not a legally valid witness," declares the bureaucrat. I notice that Manuel's daughter does not translate this. She keeps her hands still.

. . .

A FEW DAYS earlier, I chatted with a local activist as we left a community roundtable. I knew from his comments during the meeting that he was searching for his mother and two brothers and fiercely supported exhumations. But as we stood by the door, he pointedly remarked, "Exhumations are very expensive." Then he said, "There is no money to pay teachers in schools here." The highlands of Guatemala are among the poorest parts of a poor country. The poverty in El Quiché is deep, and it is not accidental. Thirty-six years of armed conflict preceded by five hundred years of occupation and dispossession have left communities struggling for economic survival. The armed conflict made things harder because, in addition to massacres, the military destroyed homes and livestock and forced people off the parcels of land that their families had managed to hold on to. The genocidal strategy targeted Maya communities and culture.

When the military burned the milpa, they sought to starve people by destroying a staple crop but also to desecrate maize, which is a holy substance. Corn is life. The Popol Vuh, the sacred text of the Maya, tells of how humans were formed from corn, the primordial mother-fathers kneaded into being from yellow and white maize. The first people were created from maize, all Maya people are sustained by maize, grains of maize are passed down in families linking generations, and, traditionally, when people died, they were buried with maize in their mouths.

Since the Spanish occupation, Maya communities have been dispossessed of their lands through measures that have been blatant at times and inconspicuous at others: laws and intimidation, encroachment and extortion. In the nineteenth century, wealthy landowners and the government led a "massive assault" on Maya lands, rapacious for profits from bananas and coffee. In the twentieth century, Maya land was expropriated for projects such as industrial agriculture and hydroelectric dams. Struggles for land continue in the twenty-first century, fueled by mining claims, tourism, and conservation projects. Maya K'iche' sociologist Gladys Tzul Tzul tells of how in the early 2000s, women were digging in the ground, searching for the bones of people killed in the genocide, when they discovered employees of a mining company "looking under the same earth for minerals." Past and present struggles converge in "the land where the dead rest and water is born."

. . .

WHEN I ACCOMPANY forensic team members to local hamlets to record oral histories and collect DNA samples, stories of genocidal violence play out against the backdrop of structural violence—the harms inflicted by a society's failure to meet people's basic needs, like food, shelter, and education. We spend all day crisscrossing the rugged terrain of El Quiché to visit three local families. These trips are necessary because many families searching for disappeared relatives cannot afford to travel for DNA tests, even if the tests themselves are free. It costs a day's wages just to take a bus to the capital to file papers, attend a hearing, or get a cheek swab. Justice is expensive.

At our first stop, we meet with Don Nico, who is thirty-nine and hardscrabble thin. He tells us that his father disappeared on his way home from a job picking coffee. Work on coffee and banana plantations is notoriously difficult and low-paying. Workers describe it as "hateful," "abhorrent," and not a form of work but of "sufrimiento" (suffering); a place where you get malaria and don't get paid. We sit in the yard of Don Nico's house, a single room with a dirt floor and a firepit in the corner. His three-year-old son plays with a plastic bag and two sticks, sniffling with a cold. As we talk, Don Nico quietly transforms the bag into a little kite, and his son races around the yard, making it fly.

The second visit is high in the hills, where Doña Vilma, who is seventy, reports the disappearance of her father, mother, and brother. She invites us into her one-room house, where the floor is ridged with boot tracks imprinted in dried mud. Her furniture is propped on bricks and chunks of wood to keep it dry. The ceiling and walls don't meet, and rain pours through the gaps where today we catch glimpses of blue sky. She loads our hands with flower bulbs and yerba buena as we leave.

Our final stop is off the main road. We cross a plank laid over a ditch to meet Don Juan and Doña Inez, a frail couple in their seventies. Sitting on chunks of firewood in their yard, they tell us about losing two sons, ages fourteen and seventeen, taken by soldiers two weeks apart and never seen again. Their surviving children have left because they cannot earn a living locally. It begins to rain, and the ditch swells with pestilent water as we leave. I think of Doña Vilma, her floor turning to mud in the downpour.

Adequate housing and food; safe drinking water and decent sanitation; access to medical care and education—these are human rights recognized by international bodies, and they are in short supply for many survivors of La Violencia. Reflecting on the proliferation of mass graves around the world, anthropologist and physician Paul Farmer writes, "What do all of these victims have in common? Not language or gender or political views; not religion or race or ethnicity. What they share, all of them, is poverty and, generally, an unwillingness to knuckle under." Maya activists have organized to demand reparations for the genocide. Unwilling to knuckle under, they seek commitments from the government to build houses, schools, and hospitals in Maya communities. They have won important battles, including a national reparations program. But, as anthropologist Irma Alicia Velásquez Nimatuj argues, "when we talk about reparations in the Guatemalan context, these often include commitments that should already be the responsibility of the state"—essential services that people like Doña Vilma need.

That Manuel cannot read is a matter not unconnected to his mother's death, to why we are standing in the Ministry, looking at the plastic sandals that did not carry her to safety. Violence is both swift and slow. It brutally erupts—soldiers shooting a mother and son as they run across a field. And it grinds down and rots away—towns without medical clinics, schools without teachers, children without enough nourishing food, grandmothers without a decent roof over their heads. Like bullet holes and machete blows, the marks of poverty can be seen on skeletons, in poorly healed fractures and rotten teeth, in the small stature of malnourishment. The marks of structural violence often accompany the marks of apocalyptic violence.

. . .

ENRAGED THAT MANUEL has been a witness to the state's genocide yet cannot be a witness on its paperwork, I want to call someone to report the bureaucrat. This useless, silly impulse rises and pops like a bubble—all phone lines lead to his office. He is the "someone," the only one that matters. His whim will rule. Alvaro, unfailingly polite, urges him to call Guatemala City again. After another hour and more phone calls, the bureaucrat inexplicably relents just before lunchtime. He signs the papers to release the bodies. He says that Manuel should be grateful; he is doing the family a favor.

. . .

CARLOS FROM THE team pulls the pickup truck in front of the Ministry, and Alvaro and Manuel load the boxes of bones and clothes into the bed, hurrying as if the bureaucrat might change his mind. Manuel and his daughter climb into the back. Family and friends follow, piling in around the boxes. Despite the tragic cargo, there is a sense of triumph as we drive away. To celebrate our victory at the Ministry, Alvaro stops to buy sweet tortillas from a woman grilling them by the side of the road. We pass the sispaque around the truck, everyone gleefully breaking off hot pieces and discussing the different names for this treat and the many words for "new corn." We speed along the road, through the green corridor of milpa, past the village with two white churches, left at the pink house, up a steep and rutted road toward the family's compound.

The floor of the three-room cement-block house is thickly spread with pine needles. A table is laden with flowers, candles, and a picture of La Virgen. Fragrant smoke billows from a bowl of copal incense. Alvaro, Carlos, and three young men from the family set the boxes on the table. There are also two empty wooden boxes I hadn't noticed before, coffins of sorts, but much smaller. Women gather to fuss with the flowers and candles. Soon the room is crowded with people. As we stand shoulder to shoulder, Don Isidoro, an uncle from a nearby village, makes a short speech, declaring this to be an important day and thanking the team for the return of Doña Asunción and Oscar. He begins to pray. Suddenly everyone is praying out loud, each in their own cadence, in Ixil and Spanish. Above the web of sound, Don Isidoro preaches Señor and Jesus. The prayer lasts fifteen minutes or longer; I lose track of time. The crowd, the smoke, the chanting, and the presence of the bodies are dizzying.

In Manuel's family, as with many Guatemalan families, people practice different faiths in different ways. Some are Catholic, and some have converted to Evangelical Christianity, which has a powerful presence in the country. Some follow costumbre, the Maya Cosmovision in which humans and the natural world are interwoven, tied to sacred maize and the spirits of the mountains. Many people combine aspects of costumbre, Catholicism, and Evangelicalism as in this ceremony.

⸱ ⸱ ⸱

DURING THE ARMED conflict, religious differences were often political dividing lines. Ríos Montt was a fervent Evangelical and supported by many of his faith, whereas Catholicism was more likely to be associated with guerrilla movements and Maya land rights struggles. In some massacres, Catholics were singled out. Maya religious practices and cultural traditions were targeted as part of the genocidal attempt to systematically eradicate Indigenous cultures. Ríos Montt established "model villages" where families displaced by the violence were forced to live under constant surveillance, and where the military sought to enforce cultural assimilation through policies such as requiring the use of the Spanish language.

After the genocide, communities divided by violence began to come together to rebuild and seek justice. People from different villages, speaking different languages and practicing different religions, worked for common goals with a strong sense of shared Maya identity.

· · ·

WHEN THE PRAYER ends, Zulma produces a piece of plain white cloth with raw edges; Alvaro opens the lid of one of the wooden boxes and drapes the fabric inside the little coffin. Carlos opens the cardboard box containing the remains of Doña Asunción. Her bones are in the same brown paper bags used in the lab, labeled with identifying codes and osteological terms: right femur, left humerus, and so on. Carlos hands Alvaro a bag, and he begins carefully fitting one vertebra to the next.

I am surprised by this sight. I did not expect the boxes to be opened and the bones publicly exhibited, much less articulated. It goes against some sense I have that remains are private, but here they are exposed for all to see. Manuel and his daughter stand to the side, watching intently. Family members hand Alvaro a new red corte, a traditional skirt, and a huipil with a simple embroidered border. Having articulated the spine, he slides it under the blouse. He calls for each bone by name. He slips a humerus into the sleeve, arranging the radius and ulna as if her arms were by her side. He continues like this until her body is pieced together, but in compacted form, the bones stacked to fit in the small box. Watching Alvaro with Doña Asunción's bones, I am struck by this meeting of science and ritual and the juxtaposition of care and clinical detachment. He arranges the bones almost tenderly but calls them by their Latin names. He touches them gently but with latex-gloved hands.

In the corner of the room, two older women lean on each other, crying, visibly grief-stricken. Everyone else seems mostly curious. A group of children pushes to the front of the crowd. They glance back at their mothers and aunts, pointing to their own legs and arms, confirming that this is where the bones come from.

Finally, Alvaro places the cranium in the box. Doña Asunción's granddaughter hands him a new bandanna, and he ties it around the skull. The dressed skeleton is, for me, a disturbing sight. I don't sense that others in the crowded room feel the same. I find myself asking forgiveness, from whom I am not sure, Manuel perhaps, or Doña Asunción herself, for my reaction.

Alvaro begins the process of arranging Oscar's bones. The family hands him a new T-shirt and a pair of puffy sweatpants. The kids watching at the front of the crowd wear the same things, but hand-me-downs. The garments are small. Oscar was a little boy. When Alvaro has articulated the tiny skeleton, he knots a bandanna over Oscar's fractured skull. He pauses to explain that it was not a bullet that caused the damage but the weight of the earth from burial—children's bones are fragile. Relief palpably ripples through the crowd that the broken skull is not a sign of violence done to the small body. With both skeletons complete, Alvaro opens the boxes of clothes, the ones strewn across the floor of the Ministry this morning. He sets a bowl and a tin cup beside Oscar's body. A woman steps forward and stops him, telling him to remove it. She explains that the cup initially buried in the hasty grave is not acceptable because it is metal. The bowl is fine because it is barro, clay, and from the earth. One of the kids is sent to find replacements, returning a few minutes later with ceramic mugs, which Alvaro nestles beside both bodies. He begins adding the old clothes. The woman stops him again. She tells him to move them so they don't cover the boy's skull. She says that the clothes cause too much pressure; "they are suffocating." Alvaro makes the adjustment, and people around me murmur in approval; yes, that's better. The ritual is as precise as the science. Just as the bones had to be placed in the correct order, so too funerals demand order, that things be done properly. Carlos extracts the final bag from the box. It holds nothing but dirt, which Alvaro pours into the corners of both boxes.

When I was cleaning skeletons in the lab, I was told to collect any soil that I brushed from bones or shook out of clothes. All this dust was carefully captured on newspapers and funneled into labeled bags. I assumed this was for some sort of sophisticated laboratory analysis, like something on *CSI*. But it was not for science. It was for the families to have some of the earth where the body of their loved one had rested.

Alvaro closes the lids of the little coffins. With a marker, he writes the forensic case identification numbers on their wood flanks. At the urging of the family, he adds the names, Oscar and Doña Asunción, and draws a small cross on each lid so that everyone will know where the heads are, and they can be buried in the proper orientation. Alvaro and Carlos step away, and a group of women pours in to adjust the boxes, arrange the flowers and candles, and fan the copal incense.

· · ·

INHUMATIONS REQUIRE RITUAL creativity. They are similar to funerals but not the same because the remains are returned to families and communities long after death. Anthropologists have

long considered funerals to be among the most stable and enduring rituals. The ways of the dead are slow to change. But catastrophic violence can bring new forms of death rituals out of
necessity. In the United States, the Civil War changed American
funerals. Families wanted to bury their fathers and sons at home,
and embalming was developed to preserve the bodies of soldiers
killed in the South until they could be brought to families in the
North. What started as a scientific solution to the problem of
shipping cadavers on trains became a standard part of American
funerals.

Rituals may seem, by definition, to be unchanging, but even
the most abiding traditions can evolve through reworking, bor-
rowing, and inventing. Arranging the bones in anatomical order,
as Alvaro has done with the remains of Doña Asunción and
Oscar, isn't necessary from a scientific point of view after analysis in the lab. It isn't something done in a traditional funeral,
where the body is fleshed and whole. But it is done at many inhumations where the team, family, and community work together,
combining elements of forensics and funerals to create something new. Placing the bones in order becomes part of the ritual
that moves bones from matter to meaning, like cups and blankets for the afterlife.

．．．

AFTER THE CEREMONY, Zulma addresses a group of about a
dozen women sitting on a narrow wooden bench against the
wall. "Who would like to share their testimonio with the North
American anthropologist?" she asks in Spanish and Ixil. Zulma
pushes a young woman named Laura, who is training as a translator, to stand by me. Laura looks nervous. She wrings her hands
in front of her corte. I'm uncomfortable, too: It seems intrusive
to record testimonios during such an intimate event, but Zulma

insists that it will be good to do. She pulls a straight-backed chair to the center of the room and gestures for me to sit.

"Come. Tell your story. She is writing a book."

Don Jaime said to me, "The world must not forget what happened here." But sharing with me is not sharing with the world. Half a dozen people came to the last conference talk I gave, and even big-name anthropologists aren't widely read outside the field. These stories will help my research—but how will it benefit these women? It seems terribly wrong, and thoughts like these are slowly eating away at my relationship with anthropology.

But I have no time to analyze my thoughts or pull apart the threads of the knot in my stomach because Zulma has pulled a second chair into place, facing me, and is saying, "The important thing is that we share what happened to us with those who are too young to remember." There is a murmur of agreement among the women. Manuel's daughter is sent out of the room and returns a few minutes later with a large group of older children. The kids stand at the door, passing pink and green lollipops back and forth.

. . .

MEMORY IS A battleground in Guatemala. During high-profile human rights trials in 2013, public buses were plastered with signs paid for by politicians that read NO HUBO GENOCIDIO (There was no genocide), while signs on other buses proclaimed SÍ HUBO GENOCIDIO (Yes, there was genocide).

. . .

ZULMA USHERS DOÑA Solana forward from the bench. I recognize her as one of the women weeping during the ceremony. Manuel and his daughter move close. Doña Solana begins her testimonio by telling us she was with Doña Asunción in a group of people trying to escape to hide in the mountains. "She was pregnant," Laura translates from Ixil to Spanish. Doña Solana says, "There were many shots." She pulls her arms tightly across her body. "Shots from the army." Her voice catches, and she begins crying. She is having a hard time finishing her sentence through her tears. Laura stops translating. For a minute, she stands in silence, then she turns to Zulma and me and says quietly in Spanish, "Talking about this is making her very sad. We should stop."

I wonder if she is right. Is this doing more harm than good? The children watch intently, waiting to see what will happen. Zulma says to Laura, "Ask her if she wants to continue." Laura asks, and Doña Solana's reaction needs no translation; she wants to go on. Zulma says, clearly addressing everyone, "It is good to take the lid off sadness."

. . .

A TESTIMONIO IS a personal story about an experience of political violence, but it is more than that. It works on several levels: part activism, part oral history, part therapy. As a form of political testimony, it seeks justice, even when it can't be found in courts. It is a public witness stand. As a form of reflection, it ties together personal and community suffering and creates space to make sense of painful experiences; it "takes the lid off sadness," as Zulma said.

It took time for me to understand what might be cooking in the pot of testimonio. I was a graduate student of anthropology, parachuting in from a North American university, a white woman among Ixil Maya women my mother's and grandmother's ages. Their stories described experiences of danger, loss, and violence beyond anything I could imagine, having lived a life of safety.

Earlier, when we arrived at the house and were eating lunch,

Alvaro took the first bite of tortilla and said, "Hmm." Zulma said, "The corn isn't from here," furrowing her brow. I chewed slowly, trying to taste what the others did. I could not. To those with sensitivity to detect it, the tortillas tasted like struggle, of having to buy inferior corn at the market rather than growing it on ancestral land. Just as I couldn't taste the corn, there were many things I didn't understand.

I thought I was supposed to be doing the ethnographic interviews I had been trained to conduct in my methods class that met on Wednesday afternoons in a seminar room overlooking a manicured lawn. But real life is not a campus, and a testimonio is not an interview. It is on the storyteller's terms. The listener is not passive—the listener is ethically implicated. Anyone hearing a testimonio is changed by it. The acidic thoughts about anthropology percolating in my mind and my discomfort sitting in that straight-backed chair in the center of the room were signs that testimonio had begun its work on me.

I was slowly learning that the soup pot of testimonio contains many ingredients: silence and words, the need to remember and the need to keep moving forward, a reckoning with the past and a demand for the future. Stirred with care, temperature modulated (lid on, lid off), testimonio can nourish the teller and the listener, family and community—and, maybe, change the world.

．．．

DOÑA SOLANA BEGINS to speak again, her voice assertive, and Laura translates: "They ran. Doña Asunción was running. She fell—" Before she can finish the sentence, Manuel interrupts. He urgently signs to his daughter, who says, "She fell! She fell on a rock!" He signs again, "Her stomach exploded." Horror stills the air. The terror of the mother. The pain of the son. The women on the bench turn to look at the two boxes, the small coffins. The children summoned for the testimonios stop fidgeting and follow their gaze. Testimonio has brought Doña Asunción and Oscar into the room as vividly as witnessing their bones.

.   .   .

LATE IN THE afternoon, the circle of testimonios breaks open. Women are still telling their stories, but around them, the day has turned into a party, festive and restless. A radio plays bachata, crackling in and out of reception. Bottles of beer and something stronger are passed around. A group of children ask to borrow my camera and run off with it, returning at intervals to show me photos of themselves clowning in the yard.

Two uncles pull their chairs to the edge of the testimonios, drinking with grim determination. Every now and then, they step into the circle to deliver pronouncements:

These murderers got away with everything.

These men with bloody hands.

These men are in power still.

We have to hear their names on the radio every day.

Ríos Montt. Lucas García. Otto Pérez, the one they call Tito.

People crowd into the room, milling around, interjecting their own memories. Stories intertwine and interrupt one another. As the testimonios lose their structure and fall apart at the edges, there are glimpses of suffering and terror.

I had no milk. Nothing to give my children.

They even burned the milpa.

There was no salt. Nothing to make tortillas. One little spoon of salt cost a quetzal.

Thank God for the rocks! We hid behind the rocks!

We were sad and in pain then.

Now we are still sad and in pain!

The room is a dissonant chorus, like the earlier prayer. In traditional Ixil funerals, four elders lead four different prayers simultaneously, converging on meaningful phrases with an artistry that linguistic anthropologist María Luz García compares to the complex patterns of Ixil Maya weaving. García has analyzed formal prayers recited at inhumations and found that they maintain this traditional funeral form but add new references to La Violencia. She notes that "blankets and clothes" and "corn and salt" are mentioned in pairs to express the hardships of the time. She gives the example of a prayer that says: "They had no clothes. They had no blankets. They had no salt."

Around me, the women giving testimonios, the people jumping in with their stories, and the uncles interjecting political commentary aren't offering formal prayers. But the form—words diverging and harmonizing—and the content—descriptions of suffering told in corn and salt—seem to borrow from traditional prayers. Around me, what is being offered is perhaps best captured by another funeral ritual, which appears in many cultures: lament. An ancient form of expressing grief through song and story, lamentation allows mourners "to honour and appease the dead" and "give expression to a wide range of conflicting emotions." Inhumations are giving rise to new forms of funeral rituals created by necessity. Through articulating skeletons and dressing the bones in new clothes, through furnishing blankets and cups for death's journey, in testimonios, stories, and political outrage, Doña Asunción and Oscar are honored and lamented.

. . .

THE ROOM IS so smoky now that I cannot see the far wall. I have escaped the chair and sit on a bench next to Zulma. Someone hands us plastic cups of sugary coffee. Suddenly, Manuel steps into the center of the room. The crowd goes quiet. He takes a photograph out of his pocket and holds it like a pledge, turning slowly, showing it to everyone gathered. It is a photo of his mother with her two sons. Elegantly dressed, her hair braided in ribbons and wrapped like a crown around her head, Doña Asunción looks straight into the camera. Manuel signs to his daughter emphatically, and she translates reluctantly. He says that he has lost his mother and brother. He has lost their village and their land. He is the only son who survived and he has been left to try to farm a rocky milpa where corn is hard to grow. The bodies of his mother and brother have been returned, and that is good. But he has one thing to ask: Is there any compensation for all he has lost? Is there any help?

"I am poor," says Manuel.

CHAPTER 5

Día de los Muertos

AN ENORMOUS RED Coca-Cola banner strung across the main gate says WELCOME TO THE GENERAL CEMETERY. Two giant inflatable Coke bottles stand sentry at the entrance. Inside, more branded bunting and flags wave in the wind. I glimpsed a headline a few days ago announcing that drinking soda might be as bad for you as smoking cigarettes, so I have to wonder about this marketing campaign.

It is the Day of the Dead, and the atmosphere at Guatemala City's historic public cemetery is celebratory. A man on a yellow bicycle sells hot dogs, and another man carries a ten-foot pole strung with cotton candy. A mariachi band wanders between the graves. Women sitting on the curb sell bouquets of chrysanthemums and strands of marigolds, known as flor de muerto. The cemetery is festive, but a subtle undercurrent of menace hums below. A crowd presses around the police arresting two pickpockets, teenage boys dressed tough and looking scared. An ambulance siren wails nearby, inside the cemetery. Maxi hears gunshots in the distance and asks me if I heard them, too. He points out how many of the graves are for dead teenagers.

Death is a booming business. By the front gates of the cemetery, near the city morgue, there are dozens of funeral homes, coffin makers, and tombstone carvers. Granite dust collects in the gutters. Caskets are propped on end by the sidewalk. A pirate funeral industry thrives; entrepreneurs called "calaqueros," skull mongers, and "zopilotes," vultures, wait outside hospitals, morgues, and crime scenes to sell their wares.

Families gather around graves, cleaning and decorating. People balance on ladders to reach the top nichos. Observing three women arranging plastic daisies in the dirt, I think about how team members often say that the purpose of exhumation is so that families have a place to bring flowers.

I think of my dead. I think of the cold March morning I walked across the parking lot of a funeral home a few towns over—the big town where the Greyhound bus stops. It had begun to snow, and plows rumbled by on the highway. This is where my father's ashes had been delivered from the crematorium. It was a utilitarian building with vinyl siding and a new roof. It looked like an insurance office or a lumberyard. I swung open the glass door, signed a few papers, and a few minutes later, they handed me a square blue cardboard box.

I was astounded that a man could be reduced to something so small. The word "ash" is light, but the box was heavy. The weight of the package was not proportional to its size, and its density and heft felt dangerous, like an explosive device. And so it was— the bomb blast of his death blew me apart. I have thought of that blue box often in Guatemala. What it means to multiply that blast by the factor of a massacre. What it means that the men who wired the bombs and lit the fuses live in impunity. How a mass grave is a megaton detonation of grief. An impact crater of loss.

. . .

YESTERDAY, AT THE lab, we talked about what people were doing for the Day of the Dead. Julia, who had just returned from the field, said she would make a platter of cured meats and pickled vegetables, a special dish for the celebration called "fiambre," with a double meaning of "cold cuts" and "corpse." I have the impulse to tell my dad; he would find it funny, but where do you send a joke to the dead? Dark humor trails the dead through morgues and labs and through this festival, too, with its dancing skeletons and wordplay. Rafa, one of the newest members of the team, said he would build an altar to the people in his family who have passed away—this is the tradition, along with cleaning the house, visiting graves, and building a path from the house to the cemetery so the dead can find their way. I am unsettled by the idea that the dead get lost.

I was visiting my father when I died. He was living far down a dirt road in an uninsulated cabin someone was letting him use. He spent his time stoking the woodstove and sitting at the kitchen table sketching still lifes and filling out employment applications. The latter activity was a requirement of his probation. He didn't want their jobs, and he told me the trick was to apply only for positions you aren't qualified to do. He also had to get drug tested weekly. He hadn't worked out a trick for this yet. He said what surprised him most about sobriety was his dreams: They were vivid, in Technicolor.

I had an asthma attack. I didn't go to the hospital because I didn't have insurance. I thought I could wait it out, and by the time I realized I couldn't, it was too late. The car was broken down. The ambulance had trouble on the bad road. Dying was easy. A moment of panic when I could not take a breath, then calm. I remember the silence in my body when my heart stopped, like a room when the electricity goes out.

I woke up in the hospital covered in vomit and shit. "The medics had to revive you twice in the ambulance," the nurse told me. It was a scolding. She told me I should have come to the hospital sooner. She said I was lucky to be alive but did not help me clean up.

My father arrived with a change of clothes. Flushed and fevered, he told me about how he'd done CPR until the ambulance came. He was amazed how it came back to him. With manic energy, he said we'd make a jailbreak. The nurse made him sign a form, overenunciating the words "against medical advice." My father's front tooth was missing. I wanted to tell the nurse that it hadn't always been missing. It could be fixed. But I didn't say anything; I was weak. My chest and ribs hurt. I was holding a plastic bag of my shitty clothes on my lap. My father signed the paper without reading it. We drove home in a borrowed car, radio on, windows open even though it was cold, with a feeling of freedom and conspiracy. I had cheated death. My father respected nothing more than getting away with something, beating the system.

I was seventeen when my father saved my life, and seventeen years later, he died: 17/17 like the double-patterned wings of a moth. This fearful symmetry feels like a clue but is probably just our cognitive condition, our human pattern-seeking.

The night my father died, my brother had a dream about him. He said, "I'm going away. Don't burn down the house." This was just what he would say. He was funny. He once told me he was his probation officer's favorite, and it's probably true. He was charming. He was difficult. He was dead.

By the time I got a flight home and drove through the snow to his house, his body had been taken away. We found a note on his table, among his sketches. "No autopsy" was all it said. This note troubled me for years. Did he want to die, or did he just know that he was dying? An autopsy report might have answered this question, but I did not seek it out. If it existed, it would mean that we had failed him. I wanted him to have his modest dying wish. I didn't want anything to happen to his body. His beautiful gardener's hands, his warm back that, as a child, I liked to place my cheek against to listen to his breath and the drum of his voice.

The absence of my father's body, the note, the autopsy that probably did take place, and the box of ashes he was reduced to, stirred something in me: some primordial question about the dead.

I went back to school after he died. I felt old and sad in my seminars but fiercely grateful to be there. It was hard to believe that this, too, was a way people lived: sitting around a table talking about dense texts, windows overlooking the haze of San Francisco Bay. I worried about mispronouncing words like "hegemony" and thought about my father's advice to apply for jobs you aren't qualified to do. Maybe I had just slipped through. Mostly I spent long hours alone reading about the dead. Like a good academic, I made an intimate enigma into a research question.

. . .

IN THE MUNICIPAL cemetery, presidents are buried next to gang members. A tomb for police sits near a crypt that looks like an Egyptian monument. On its outskirts, the cemetery drops precipitously into the municipal landfill. You smell it before you see it. The jagged boundary looks unstable; the cemetery is crumbling into the dump. Dozens of vultures circle overhead. A father and son piss over the edge.

Shacks and tents line the periphery of the landfill. Garbage pickers sort through the waste. Faded plastic flowers and broken planks from caskets have been tossed over the cemetery's edge into the dump. There are dozens of bones, but they aren't human; they are from the vultures. Maxi says that gangs dump their victims in the landfill. I remember hearing that one of the teaching skeletons in the lab had been found here. I think of how survivors told Jesuit priest and anthropologist Ricardo Falla that after a massacre in Huehuetenango the earth had been "blackened with vultures."

At the entrance of the cemetery, next to a Coca-Cola sign saying OPEN HAPPINESS, a stark banner gives instructions regarding OVERDUE PUBLIC NICHOS, advising SETTLE YOUR PAYMENTS; OTHERWISE, THE EXHUMATION PROCESS WILL BEGIN, signed THE ADMINISTRATION. The cemetery has run out of space, and bodies are aggressively removed to make room. Failure to pay for a grave or a nicho results in quick removal of the dead.

A nicho costs Q200 (25 USD), with payments due every four years. If the fees aren't paid, cemetery workers hammer open the grave or nicho. They bundle the remains in a plastic bag and deposit them in the cemetery's ossuary, a deep dry well of bones. Everything else, clothing, coffin, plastic flowers, is tossed into the landfill.

Maxi paces nearby, making a call. I take a photograph of the vultures perched on top of the ice-cream-colored nichos. Nearby, a group of boys fly kites. In some parts of Guatemala, flying kites on Día de los Muertos is a tradition to communicate with the dead. At the edge of the cemetery, the boys let out their spools of string; as they unravel, the wind pulls the kites higher and higher until they dip and swoop with the vultures.

CHAPTER 4

An Archive of Surveillance

I N JULY 2005, investigators entered a sprawling police compound in Zone 6 of Guatemala City looking for explosives. Three weeks earlier, at the nearby Mariscal Zavala military base, a stockpile of weapons left over from the armed conflict had detonated, showering debris on residential neighborhoods and forcing mass evacuations. Looking to avert a similar catastrophe, investigators searched the vast grounds, which contained barracks, an abandoned hospital, a wrecking yard of junked cars, and a canine training unit. They discovered munitions but also found something arguably more explosive: a hidden archive belonging to the National Police—an immense record of human rights abuses.

The word "archive" elicits visions of pristine, alphabetized libraries and temperature-controlled storage, but investigators found piles of papers festering where they'd been dumped in a half-constructed building. An estimated eighty million pages detailing surveillance, torture, and disappearance teetered in stacks, some ten feet high. Folders labeled "assassinations" and "kidnappings" packed rusty file cabinets. A *New York Times* reporter who gained access to the archive four months after its discovery described it as "staring down a tidal wave." Infested with cockroaches and sprouting fluorescent mildew, it would prove to be the largest secret cache of state documents in the history of Latin America.

So began an improbable project to recuperate what came to be known as the Historical Archives of the National Police. Launched in times of impunity, it was staffed by human rights activists and headed by Gustavo Meoño Brenner, a former national leader in Ejército Guerrillero de los Pobres, the Guerrilla Army of the Poor. By a twist of fate, the activists once targeted in the archive's files came to be in charge of poring through its secrets.

Alberto Fuentes Rosales, the project coordinator, tells us, "These kinds of things only happen in Guatemala and Macondo," referring to the town in Gabriel García Márquez's *One Hundred Years of Solitude.* There are strange and magical details to the story. Some documents survived because rain blowing in through the broken windows soaked the top layer of the pile, creating a papier-mâché shell that protected the papers underneath. In 2007, a giant sinkhole appeared in the neighborhood, swallowing a city block but sparing the archive.

More than magic, the archive is labor. Around us, a hive of staff members wearing caps, gloves, and masks clean documents with soft-bristled brushes, pull out rusty staples, and wrap neat parcels in acid-free paper. Several rooms are dedicated to storing processed documents. Like exhumed bones, the sorted papers wait in coded boxes stacked to the ceiling. International donors fund the project, recognizing the importance of the archive in the quest for accountability and justice. The documents are digitally preserved by institutions outside of Guatemala in case anything happens to the physical copies, a necessary precaution because the building has been attacked with Molotov cocktails, and archivists have received death threats. Archivists press pages to the glass surface of the industrial scanner, digitizing to its constant hum and ecliptic light. They have been organizing, preserving, and cataloging the documents for a decade; they have a long way to go.

· · ·

GUATEMALAN WRITER RODRIGO Rey Rosa describes the police archive as "a kind of micro-chaos, the telling of which could serve as a coda for the singular danse macabre of our last century." The contemporary chapter of Guatemala's troubles began in 1954 when the U.S. government sponsored the overthrow of the democratically elected, left-leaning president Jacobo Árbenz Guzmán. The coup d'état was carried out in the name of fighting Communism and protecting the interests of the colossal American corporation the United Fruit Company (later Chiquita Brands), whose profits were threatened by Árbenz's land-reform policies. The coup sparked one of the longest conflicts in Central American history, a region notable for its intransigent political struggles. Thirty-six years of violence and terror followed.

From the beginning, the United States funded and advised Guatemala's authoritarian governments. Green Beret and CIA advisers coached the military on brutal counterinsurgency tactics, and Guatemalan military commanders were trained at the U.S. Army–directed School of the Americas. In the 1980s, the United States maintained close ties with the Guatemalan government as the Guatemalan military committed genocide.

The violence reached an apex between 1981 and 1983, notably during the government of General Efraín Ríos Montt, whose ties to the United States were particularly close. He graduated from an officer-training institute "that would eventually be known as the School of the Americas," and later learned counterinsurgency tactics at Fort Bragg, North Carolina. He served as a head of department at the Inter-American Defense College in Washington, D.C. He became an Evangelical preacher at a Guatemalan church affiliated with a Pentecostal mission based in California. He was praised by Ronald Reagan and admired by Pat Robertson and Jerry Falwell. His daughter, Zury Ríos Sosa, an influential Guatemalan political figure in her own right who made a bid for the presidency in 2015, is married to Jerry Weller, former U.S. representative for Illinois's Eleventh Congressional District.

General Ríos Montt wrought apocalyptic violence on Guatemala. Under plans like "Fusiles y Frijoles" (rifles and beans), his government pursued a "scorched earth" policy of destroying villages, burning crops, displacing people, and slaughtering civilians. In the first five months of Ríos Montt's tenure, the military killed more than ten thousand people. Like Guatemalan dictators before and after him, Ríos Montt targeted rural Maya communities for their perceived support of guerrilla groups, proclaiming his aim to "drain the water where the fish swim."

· · ·

TRUTH COMMISSIONS, INTERNATIONAL judiciaries, and national courts have recognized the violence in Guatemala as genocide. Yet the politicians and military leaders responsible have faced little consequence. Many in power at the height of the violence have gone on to have long, illustrious careers, holding top government posts, including presidencies. Against this tide of impunity, General Ríos Montt was convicted of crimes against humanity and genocide in 2013. It was a stunning victory: Ríos Montt was the first former head of state to be found guilty of genocide in their own country.

Ten days later, judges overturned the conviction on a technicality. After the trial, Ríos Montt continued to live in a comfortable suburb of Guatemala City, where he died at home in April 2018. He was ninety-one—ninety years older than the child whose skull I tried to piece together in the FAFG lab, one small body found in a large mass grave dating to Ríos Montt's presidency.

• • •

LA VERBENA CEMETERY is "the epicenter of the search for the disappeared" in Guatemala City. There, the Guatemalan forensic team is searching for bodies of the disappeared that were dumped into ossuaries—deep, circular pits where bones removed from graves and nichos to make room for the more recently dead are unceremoniously deposited. They are also known as "bone wells," which is a better description. The exhumation takes place in a far corner of the cemetery. The team works inside a semi-open structure with cement-block walls and a corrugated metal roof, a much more permanent arrangement than the tarps and tents of most excavations. Pilar, who has worked here since the project began, greets us, standing among hundreds of clear plastic bags filled with bones and bodies. She tells us they find loose bones, complete skeletons, and bodies that have mummified and saponified. She explains the triage system: bodies with obvious trauma, like gunshot wounds, are prioritized for analysis. The team writes up case notes. One report reads:

FAFG case #1200-2776. Sex—Male, between 33-57 years of age. Skeleton—semi-complete, displaying multiple traumas, all perimortem—at the time of death. Thorax— three broken ribs on right side of rib cage. Top two left thoracic ribs broken, left scapula fractured, consistent with a crushing of the chest cavity. Left arm—missing beneath the upper quarter of the humerus, wound consistent with a high velocity projectile impact. Right foot—missing, likely amputated, perimortem. Cranium— present, with posterior trauma to the base of the skull. Massive trauma to the orbital ridge, which is missing, along with nearly all of the nasal cavity. Trauma is consistent with high velocity projectile impact, laterally, and likely the cause of death. Recovered with one white dress shirt, and one t-shirt displaying a "Puma" logo.

The team counts skulls, maxillae, and left femurs to establish the minimum number of individuals in the ossuary, which they estimate at sixteen thousand.

Pilar opens the metal trapdoor in the concrete floor. The hole releases a waft of putrid air. Hundreds of cockroaches scuttle toward the depths, where a tangle of bones, clothing, and plastic bags float in a watery scum. The bone wells are like the police archives when they were first discovered—but the moldering jumble is bodies, not papers. While the military carried out massacres in rural Guatemala, the National Police undertook campaigns of disappearance in urban areas. They targeted journalists, union members, university students, activists, militants, and others. The police abducted those they labeled "communists," "subversives," and "internal enemies," detaining their victims in secret prisons.

Deep in the labyrinth of the police archive, there is a walled-off area with cells where people were imprisoned, tortured, and killed.

Before the documents were dumped here, the building was a clandestine detention center known as La Isla. The human rights violations of the National Police were so grave that it was dismantled as part of the peace accords in 1996 and replaced by the National Civil Police. Sometime afterward, the archives were hidden in the compound in Zone 6.

The term "disappearance" was coined in Guatemala and made infamous during Argentina's dictatorship, but the practice was first introduced by Nazis in the Second World War. Adolf Hitler's Nacht und Nebel (Night and Fog) decree of 1941 was designed to make prisoners "vanish without leaving a trace" and "leave the family and the population uncertain as to the fate" of the missing. At the Nuremberg trials, the Night and Fog disappearances were recognized as a fundamental innovation in war crimes, notable for their extreme cruelty toward prisoners and their families and loved ones. Enforced disappearance was recognized as a crime against humanity in the 1998 Rome Statute of the International Criminal Court.

. . .

IN GUATEMALA, THE bodies of the disappeared were burned, hidden in mass graves, buried without names in urban cemeteries, dumped in ossuaries, and sometimes thrown in volcanoes. Families and friends searched for the missing, not knowing if they were alive or dead. Guiding us through the archive, Fuentes tells us, "They took away our right to life, but they also took away our right to death." He stops by an open box and pulls out a "ficha," an index card typed with a man's name, five dates, and a scribbled note. He extracts a logbook and pries open its water-damaged cover to reveal row after row of photos glued in place. Most aren't mugshots. People look brightly into the camera: hair combed, wearing lipstick and jewelry, ties and shirt collars tidy. Some smile. These are pictures from driver's licenses and ID cards, appropriated to track "delinquents" and "subversives."

The extent of the surveillance is apparent in the thousands of fichas and annotated lists of names with captions like "security measures," "subject to investigation," "agitator," "subversive activities," and "guerrilla fighter." Some bear an ominous red X, and some are marked "300," a code for assassination.

Among the files discovered rotting in the archive was a folder labeled "Myrna Mack Chang." An anthropologist trained in Great Britain, Mack came home to Guatemala in 1982 at the height of La Violencia. She wanted to document what was happening in her country, but research was a perilous proposition. "Talented, spirited, and audacious" is how her collaborator, social scientist Elizabeth Oglesby, describes her. The two spent four years working together and joked that they "destroyed an entire fleet of Suzuki jeeps from the Budget Rent-A-Car office in Guatemala City" trying to reach remote villages. In photographs, Mack has a bright smile and a mischievous expression, an infectious "I dare you" look. She was among the first Guatemalan researchers to conduct fieldwork on the impact of the armed conflict on local communities in the highlands. Oglesby says, "She knew the risks of doing research in the conflict zones, especially for a Guatemalan. We were stopped and questioned on every road and path by soldiers or the army-controlled civil patrol that guarded each village." Mack often joked, "The difference between a U.S. scholar and a Guatemalan scholar, is that in the United States, you say 'Publish or perish.' Here, we say 'If we publish, we perish.'"

Mack had a "love-hate" relationship with anthropology. She loved fieldwork but hated how researchers from North America and Europe came to Latin America to devote themselves to studying "culture" stripped of politics. Anthropologists investigated topics like "ceremonial exchanges, Saint's Day rituals, weddings, baptisms, and work parties" but failed to analyze structural violence and state terror. Anthropology "diverted its gaze," in the words of anthropologist Linda Green. Mack grappled with how to do a different kind of research. In letters to friends, she wrote, "What troubles me is that all I do is talk to people. I draw out their sad histories, and that's it. I feel my role reduced to one of extraction." And, "I still wonder how to give something worth-while back."

Mack had been raised in the protected world of Guatemala's elite. She grew up riding horses, taking ballet classes, attending private schools with wealthy friends, including high-ranking military families. Through her research in remote parts of the country, she came to have a new understanding of Guatemala. She wrote, "I have seen new places where beauty and sorrow are intertwined, where there is a silent struggle to rise above pain and despair, to not surrender." Mack eventually published groundbreaking research on the aftermath of the armed conflict, documenting the ongoing impacts of state violence and forced displacement on Maya communities. On September 11, 1990, Myrna Mack was stabbed twenty-seven times and left to die on the street.

· · ·

AT THE ARCHIVE, we cross an outdoor walkway between buildings. Our guide pauses in a small garden to check on the roses, which are sparsely blooming. He stoops to search for the iguana that likes to sleep under the bushes. The staff planted the flowers because reading the files of terror day in and day out, year after year, takes a toll. Most archivists come to the work through their involvement in human rights groups; some were activists in the 1980s, and some are family members of the disappeared. It isn't unusual for the team to find files on the surveillance of family, friends, and colleagues. They need a little beauty.

· · ·

IN THE DAYS after Myrna Mack's death, the government tried to claim that she had been killed in a robbery. No one believed this. Elizabeth Oglesby remembers the call she received the morning after the murder: "They killed Myrna last night." There was no need to name the "they" in question; it was clear to everyone that she had been executed for speaking out about human rights abuses in Guatemala.

Mack's sister Helen pushed for an investigation, but she was shocked "to see how the police, judges and prosecutors didn't want to work on the case." For more than ten years, Helen relentlessly sought justice for her sister's murder, despite death threats against key witnesses, the assassination of a police investigator, and more than a dozen judges withdrawing from the case.

In 2003, the Inter-American Court of Human Rights ruled that the state assassinated Myrna Mack Chang because she brought public attention to the atrocities of La Violencia. The Guatemalan government publicly admitted responsibility for her murder a year later.

If the assassination was meant to silence Mack, it "backfired," as a Human Rights Watch report says. After Mack's murder, the human rights violations she documented gained international attention. Decades after its initial publication, her research was used as part of the expert testimonies in the trial of Ríos Montt to prove genocide. Hers is a "living and combatiente legacy," as anthropologist Diane Nelson writes, in tribute, celebrating her socially engaged research. Myrna Mack's work and life speak to the possibilities of an anthropology that refuses to divert its gaze.

. . .

To carry out political violence at scale requires organization. It requires a system. Archives are the infrastructure of what Hannah Arendt famously described as the banality of evil, which depends on filing cabinets, index cards, passport photos, fingerprints, and legions of administrative staff to staple, paste, label, and file.

The documents in the Historical Archives of the National Police trace a hundred years of state surveillance. From the 1920s, there are fingerprint cards categorized in the Vucetich system, named for the Argentine police official who first realized the potential to track people by the whorls and swirls of their fingertips. Later, under the supervision of the United States, the

Guatemalan police upgraded to the Henry classification system, originally developed by British colonial forces in India.

There are lists of names collected in the 1950s, during the years of the U.S.-backed coup to overthrow the democratically elected government, when hotels sent their guest registries to police daily to track the movements of "suspicious" visitors. Starting in the 1960s, there are photos of protesters taken with cameras provided by the U.S. Agency for International Development. In an annual report from the early 1970s, the National Police acknowledge the "valuable help" from USAID with "arms, ammunition, tear gas, special fingerprinting materials, office supplies and furniture, paint and even vehicles for the use of the different National Police Corps." From 1971, fingerprinting was no longer reserved for people detained by the police. Everyone applying for a national ID card was fingerprinted, and the archives bulged with data. The documents from the 1980s record state death squads, surveillance of activists, infiltration of unions and student groups, and codes for kidnapping and death.

"Policing is, in its most basic sense, a process by which a state builds an archive of society," observes historian Kristen Weld in her foundational book *Paper Cadavers: The Archives of Dictatorship in Guatemala.* "The work of policing—think, for example, of the criminal background check—would be impossible without the archival tools of fingerprint databases, arrest logs, and categories of circumscribed behavior." Without records and reports, there could be no blacklists, no "subversives," no detentions. Archives are tools and weapons. Among the thousands of fingerprint cards in the yellowing documents, archivists found one that, instead of inky prints, had pieces of skin stapled to the paper, like "dried rose petals."

Authoritarian governments register, track, and surveil at the same time they target, kill, and obfuscate. As a report from the Argentine forensic team notes, "The same state that was committing the crime was bureaucratically obliged, simply oblivious, or indifferent to the paper trail that it was creating."

Philosopher Jacques Derrida writes, "There is no political power without control of the archive." Once dangerous for those whose photos and fingerprints were on file, an archive can later become a liability for a state that wants to forget. Historians and journalists have drawn on the Guatemalan police archives to tell the story of state terror. Families have searched the files for information about missing relatives. Human rights groups and prosecutors have used documents to build legal cases against police and military, including abuses committed under Efraín Ríos Montt.

Archives are incompatible with political impunity, which is why they are so often hidden and destroyed. In Guatemala, during the truth commission proceedings at the end of the armed conflict, the government claimed that all relevant files had been lost or destroyed. In Argentina, when the junta left power in 1983, they ordered the destruction of military archives. In both cases, many documents survived and were later discovered. But the authoritarian state's impulse to disavow, conceal, and eradicate archives is telling. Without archives, atrocities are easier to deny. Without archives, it is easier for tyrants to whack open a "piñata of self-forgiveness" and be rewarded with what they treasure most: doubt, amnesia, and impunity.

. . .

AFTER THIRTEEN YEARS of an implausible reversal of fortune in which human rights activists took control of the evidence of state terror, the archive's luck ran out. In August 2018, the project came under systematic attack from the government of then-president Jimmy Morales. A high-profile human rights trial had recently convicted top military officials once considered "untouchable," and evidence from the archive had played an important role. Soon thereafter, the archive's longtime director, Gustavo Meoño Brenner, was dismissed, and most of the archivists were fired. In its heyday, the project had a staff of 150; it was left with just 15 employees. Access was restricted, and the government threatened legal action against the organizations outside of Guatemala hosting virtual files. When the archive was closed to the public in 2018, staff had sorted and scanned a little more than a quarter of the papers, leaving most in stacks, their secrets undiscovered. The archive's fate is uncertain.

What is certain is that archives of surveillance will continue to be amassed in Guatemala and everywhere else, even as they change form. The "history of the techniques by which states police individuals . . . includes the physiognomic techniques of the nineteenth century and the digital eavesdropping of yesterday," as Eyal Weizman, forensic investigator and founder of the field of forensic architecture, reminds us. Paper gives way to computer code, photos to facial recognition technologies, file cabinets to the cloud, logbooks to algorithms, ink on fingers to biometric scans. Surveillance expands at the same time that it becomes increasingly invisible and "frictionless." Perhaps this is why encountering the Guatemalan archive in its materiality—in its decaying immensity, like the rotting corpse of a beached whale—powerfully affected many visitors, including me. In the books filled with photos and handwritten codes that decide life and death, I glimpsed the mass surveillance that precedes mass atrocity. I saw that a ficha can be as deadly as a bullet, and how a list of names can fill a mass grave.

CHAPTER 5

Teaching Skeleton

A T THE FORENSIC LAB in Guatemala City, Nicole lifts a cranium from a box of bones. A bullet hole is clearly visible, piercing the frontal bone. "Well, there's the trauma," says Stephanie. This morning we are taking an informal test, articulating a teaching skeleton to determine sex, age, stature, and trauma without any help from Maxi.

Nicole places the cranium at the top of the table. The skull, if there is one, comes first, anchoring the rest of the bones as they are articulated. Encountering a collection of bones, anthropologists draw on systems of classification to sort them out. The axial skeleton, at the center of the body, comprises 80 bones, including the skull, vertebral column, ribs, and sternum. The appendicular skeleton, the body's extremities, is made up of 126 bones, including those of the legs (the femur, tibia, and fibula) and arms (the humerus, radius, and ulna). All skeletal elements are important for inventory and analysis. Even the smallest bones are carefully sought at exhumation sites, and soil is sieved to retrieve fragments the size of peas. But some bones play a more important role in creating a biological profile, like the skull, the pelvis, and the femur. As we examine the bones, we fill in the inventory form listing the skeletal elements, indicating which are absent and present and their condition.

Nicole stacks the ribs upside down, forming an arc, a trick to determine their anatomical order. Stephanie hands me thoracic vertebrae, and I try to align them in position from one to twelve.

I struggle to keep up with Nicole and Stephanie, who have already worked at morgues and archaeological sites and are competent and fast. I need time to examine each bone, look things up, and repeat mnemonics under my breath. For the cranial bones, "pest of six" (the six being parietal, ethmoid, sphenoid, temporal, occipital, and frontal). For carpal bones, the stalkerish "she looks too proud, try to chase her" (scaphoid, lunate, triquetrum, pisiform, trapezium, trapezoid, capitate, hamate).

The skeleton we are working on has been studied in many field schools, and its forensic profile is well known to everyone in the lab. Except us. Around us, people are quietly working, leaning over bones arrayed on tables, tapping at computers, and filling out paper forms, but we are aware that they are also watching to see how quickly and accurately we can analyze the body.

. . .

MANY OF THE remains exhumed from mass graves and articulated in the lab are never identified. This happens if there isn't sufficient evidence to match the bones to a specific missing person, like when there is no match in the DNA database or when the DNA sample is too degraded to be analyzed. On the top floor of the lab building, more than two thousand boxes of unidentified remains are kept in storage. The cardboard boxes are labeled with numbers and letters that indicate when and where they were found. One code per body. One body per box. Stacked floor to ceiling, they are packed so tightly that you have to turn sideways to squeeze between them in some places. It is a miniature city of the dead, like an architect's model of a cemetery. Instead of tree-lined boulevards with walls of nichos and rows of tombs, there are narrow paths between boxes. Instead of names and epitaphs inscribed in stone, there are Magic Marker codes. Instead of marble monuments, tilting cardboard towers.

What will happen to these bodies in boxes? Some will be returned to communities for communal burial. Most linger in limbo, awaiting identification. With each passing year, the chances get slimmer. Surviving relatives age and die before their cheek swabs are collected for the DNA database. Families move and become harder to find. Funding is directed toward more immediate projects. Bones can be preserved almost indefinitely, but time for identification runs out. Bodies in boxes wait for the past to claim them.

For bone fragments, the story is a little different. Pieces of bones found in mass graves that don't clearly belong to a particular skeleton and are too small to be genetically tested are also stored. Every year the chances of a DNA match get better because technology improves. Fragments in boxes wait for the future to claim them.

In New York, this future arrived twenty years after the September 11, 2001, attack on the World Trade Center. Stored bone fragments, once too small to yield results, were reanalyzed with cutting-edge genetic testing, leading to the identification of two people. The New York medical examiner's office consistently retests the twenty-two thousand body parts in storage with ever-more-sensitive technologies, committed to doing "whatever it takes, as long as it takes" to identify remains. The chief medical examiner called naming the dead "a sacred obligation." And while communities worldwide share this sentiment, only wealthy countries have the resources for perpetual analysis. In most places, victims' remains are stored with fading hopes of identification.

Above the lab in Guatemala City, unidentified bodies are stranded—by imperfect technology, by funding shortages, by the brutality of a genocide that scattered families and sometimes left no surviving relatives to make a DNA match. Boxes of the dead, warehouses of the dead, cities of the dead, waiting in cardboard purgatory.

• • •

THE SKELETON THAT Nicole, Stephanie, and I are piecing to-gether is one of these unidentified bodies. Teaching skeletons, like this one, are singled out for study because their profile con-tains something interesting or complex that will help forensic students like us better understand the traumas associated with mass atrocity. Reading bones is a form of hands-on knowledge that can't be gained from a textbook. It is only by working with bodies that forensic practitioners can learn to accurately assess evidence of human rights abuses.

Yet teaching skeletons themselves have a terrible human rights history. The bones and cadavers that medical students, anthropologists, and others rely on to learn subjects like anat-omy and osteology have a painful past that has yet to be fully confronted. Malevolent examples abound. In the United States in the nineteenth century, "major medical schools used slave corpses, acquired through an underground market in dead bod-ies, for education and research," as historian Daina Ramey Berry has detailed in her work. A lifetime of human rights abuses con-tinued after death, when Black people's bodies were appropri-ated for anatomical study and ultimately buried, unnamed, in mass graves.

A well-known textbook called the *Pernkopf Atlas of Topo-graphical and Applied Human Anatomy,* first published in the United States in 1963 and prized by surgeons for its detailed medical illustrations, was the work of a Nazi physician and based on dissections of the bodies of people murdered in Nazi atroci-ties. The textbook's origins only began to be questioned in the 1990s, and it remained in print until 1994.

When I was a student at the University of California, Berke-ley, I walked out of class one sunny afternoon to find protesters gathered in front of the anthropology building demanding the return of ancestral human remains. This was how I learned that UC Berkeley and the Phoebe A. Hearst Museum of Anthropology have one of the largest collections of human remains in the country, stored in the museum and under the Hearst Memorial Gymnasium swimming pool. The university retains possession of the remains of more than ten thousand individuals against the wishes of the Wiyot Tribe, Santa Rosa Rancheria Tachi Yokut Tribe, Kashia Pomo Tribe, and many other Native groups. "We don't appreciate them keeping our ancestors locked up in a drawer," Ted Howard, cultural resources director of the Shoshone-Paiute Tribes, told a reporter. "This is a human rights issue."

In the spring of 2021, journalists broke a story that human remains belonging to children were being held in storage at the University of Pennsylvania Museum of Archaeology and Anthropology. The children, believed to be twelve-year-old Delisha Africa and fourteen-year-old Tree Africa, were killed in 1985 when Philadelphia police dropped a satchel bomb on the roof of a row house on Osage Avenue, the residence of a Black liberation group known as MOVE. Six adults and five children were killed in the explosion and resulting fire, which destroyed two city blocks. In the immediate aftermath of the attack, forensic anthropologists analyzed victims' remains. But rather than being identified and returned to grieving family members, the bones were allegedly kept in storage and used by Ivy League anthropologists as teaching material for classes like Real Bones: Adventures in Forensic Anthropology.

Anthropology is grappling with these human rights abuses within the field. It has to. For forensic anthropologists and archaeologists, there is no way to escape or avoid the issue—human remains are necessary for teaching and learning. Just like medical students need to dissect cadavers to understand anatomy, forensic expertise cannot be gained without bones.

. . .

MOST STUDENTS ARE drawn to forensic exhumation work precisely for its union of science and human rights, and they care deeply about the ethical treatment of human remains. In the lab in Guatemala City, forensic training is not an academic exercise. It is essential to accurately document evidence of human rights abuses. It is integral to finding and returning the bodies of missing people to their families.

Even so, teaching skeletons can mark the edge of dangerous territory. Maxi told me that a few years previously, a student arrived at the field school with a hacksaw in her suitcase. She planned to bring home any interesting specimens of bone she found, an intention she openly announced, airily certain of her right to take anything she pleased. Naturally, Maxi set her straight. "I told her she'd do it over my dead body!" he said as he made a sawing motion over his bicep, infusing his outrage with his typical gallows humor. He confiscated her saw and informed her that such a plan was unethical and illegal.

This case is an extreme outlier. As far as I know, only one hacksaw has ever been confiscated. (And knowing Maxi, this story could be exaggerated to make a point.) Yet there is something intrinsically unsettling about students coming from around the world to study the bodies of people killed in a genocide. And we should be unsettled by it. We have to be. It is a sign that we remain ever-alert to the treatment of the dead, aware of the political and social contexts that create mass graves, and that we never forget that every set of remains is a missing person.

Maxi often says that exhumation is "destruction and recovery." He means this in an archaeological sense, that the search for bodies inevitably damages evidence. But this duality seems true in a more philosophical sense, too. Only by reckoning with the fraught history of the discipline and the destructive practices that continue in some corners of the field can forensic anthropology's full potential for human rights be recovered.

• • •

STEPHANIE PULLS A strange bone from the box. "That's not human," says Nicole.

"It's canine," says Stephanie quickly.

"I can see that," replies Nicole tartly. Their interactions are often charged with competitive voltage, which is sparking hot this morning. I feel relieved that at least I discerned that the bone looked out of place and that I wasn't completely fooled by this trick question on our forensic test.

To estimate age at death, calculate stature (height), and attribute sex, we carefully analyze the skeletal remains, examining cranial and palate suture closure, measuring femurs and metatarsals, cross-referencing our findings with decision matrices, range charts, indexes, discriminant functions, and regression equations. As we work, we consult charts and tables photocopied from textbooks, taped to the lab's walls. The photocopies we refer to have been annotated with red ink and sticky notes. Standard formulas do not always apply in Guatemala. Most were developed from narrow demographic segments—for example, the bodies of North American soldiers killed in World War II and the Korean War. These lost young men and the bodies exhumed in Guatemala do not always measure up and match, forensically speaking.

We have been warned to be cautious when using textbooks to assign categories of "probable female" or "probable male" to remains ("sexing the skeleton" in forensic parlance). In the words of one team member, "In Guatemala, female bodies will present like males." He is referring to a forensic axiom that female bones are more "gracile"—lighter and more delicate—than male bones, which are assumed to be larger and thicker. This is captured in a

2017 forensic textbook that states, "For the most part sexual dimorphism in the human skeleton can be stated as 'males are larger and more robust than females, or females are smaller and more gracile than males.'" Another textbook reads: "In sexing a skull, the initial impression is often the deciding factor, i.e., a large robust skull is generally that of a male and a small, gracile skull that of a female." But initial impressions can be misleading; they may have more to do with cultural stereotypes of graceful women and brawny men than with distinctions rooted in biology.

For one thing, hard physical labor makes bones more robust, so some forensic common sense about "sexing the skeleton" draws on gendered patterns of work rather than anything biological. In places like rural Guatemala, where women chop wood and carry water, their bones reflect these activities. Bones are also shaped by feast and famine. Nutrition influences stature. Kids who get enough to eat grow up to have larger, denser bones—something crucial to understand in places marked by structural violence and conflict.

Simplistic approaches to "sexing the skeleton" can have disastrous consequences. Studies reveal that when migrants die crossing the U.S.-Mexico border, their bodies have been misclassified using forensic formulas that fail to account for "populations that may contain smaller, gracile males." The stakes are high and forensic practitioners have to get it right or people won't be identified and their families won't know what happened to them. Recent research in forensic anthropology explores the complex interplay of biological, environmental, and social factors with more nuance. Nevertheless, old-time forensic truisms die hard.

. . .

I FIRST ENCOUNTERED the idea that culture is written in the body in a chilly lecture hall when charismatic professor Nancy

Scheper-Hughes announced to the packed medical anthropology course that our bodies are not just biological matter; they are (we are) also cultural beings. Striding across the stage, a wisp of a woman with a streak of purple in her salt-and-pepper hair and a voice that carried to the back row, she said, "We *learn* our bodies. How to swim, how to ride a bike, how to write, how to orgasm, how to nurse a baby." I had never thought of this, but I recognized its truth with a jolt.

The idea that bodies are socially, not just biologically, formed was proposed by the French sociologist Marcel Mauss in an essay called "Techniques of the Body," published in 1934. He begins by observing that the way people swim had changed since he was a boy. He was taught to swallow and spit water as he paddled, chugging along like a steamboat. "It was stupid," he writes, but even though no one swam like that anymore, he couldn't stop doing it; the habit was too deeply engrained. As a young man in World War I, he observed that the French and British troops marched differently and couldn't get the knack of marching the same way together—they only ended up looking silly when they tried. Later, as a patient in an American hospital, he noticed that the young nurses on the ward walked in a way he recognized from movies. When he returned to Paris, he was astonished to find that French women, too, had adopted this distinctive Hollywood gait. Although biology dictates that humans are bipedal, we don't all walk the same way. Our societies teach us how to march, shimmy, and swagger.

Mauss coined the termed "habitus" to describe these socially formed habits of movement. Habitus isn't just an academic theory; it is something we all know from experience. We know it from people-watching in airports: the gangly stride of Americans and the more measured European steps. We know it from taking the subway—women tightly folded in their seats and men sitting with their legs splayed (aka "manspreading"). We know it from spotting differences in social class from how someone holds their fork and knife. We learn to inhabit our bodies in specific ways, and these become deeply set, eventually no more open to alteration than changing our handwriting or the accent of our speech.

I learned about habitus in a lecture hall in California, but I didn't really understand it until I arrived at the lab in Guatemala City. Until I began to read skeletons with a forensic eye, I thought of the embodiment of culture as rather metaphorical. I didn't quite grasp that culture is materially, tangibly, written in the body.

Experienced forensic practitioners at the lab can see in the tiny bones of toes that someone was a weaver. In backstrap weaving, a technique used in Guatemala for over two thousand years and the way traditional huipils are made, the weaver kneels in front of the loom. Over time this posture causes changes ("occupational stress markers") to the back, knees, and feet, affecting the vertebrae, patellae, ischium, metatarsals, and proximal phalanges.

Tailors may develop grooves in their incisors from holding pins in their mouths as they measure and sew. Ribs can be flattened from corsets, elbows marked by walking dogs, and backs altered by carrying babies. "Milker's neck" describes compression fractures of the cervical vertebrae caused by habitually resting the head against the flank of a cow. A controversial 2018 study claimed that people may be developing a sort of horn at the back of their skull as the bone is re-formed by the habit of constantly looking down at phones. Whether or not this is true, research shows that screen time affects our bone mass. If you sit in front of a computer all day, your bones may be marked by this activity. We are the loads we carry, the looms we kneel before, the hours we spend scrolling. Life shapes us down to the bone.

· · ·

IN THE LAB, we have completed the biological profile of our teaching skeleton. We estimate that the remains are those of a "probable female" adolescent. Now we must document trauma. This would seem to be a straightforward case. It takes no special forensic training to see the bullet hole in the forehead. But like good students taking a difficult exam, Stephanie and Nicole hesitate before filling in the practice form with the obvious answer. There's a salient feature we haven't explored yet—the cranium is slightly asymmetrical, flattened on one side.

As we examine the skull, we think of the secret life of bones. Had she habitually done something that would change the shape of her head? We trade theories. In Guatemala, a common way to move bundles of firewood and other heavy things is to suspend them from a thick strap worn around the forehead. The load rests on a person's back, but their head bears the burden, too. Years of carrying things this way can remodel the skull. But the cranium isn't consistent with this shape. Perhaps it isn't life that has shaped the bone, but death.

Bones are living things. Just as breaking the trunk of a sapling is different than snapping a dry stick, living bone reacts to force differently than dead bone. Forensic texts commonly refer to living or recently dead bone as "green," as freshly cut wood is called "green," referring to its properties of resilience, not color. (In fact, living bones are pink, threaded by capillaries.) The meeting of force and bone leaves marks, and the signs are different in living and dead bone. To the trained eye, a femur crushed in a fatal accident looks different than a femur smashed years after someone's death. It is critical to be able to tell whether a torturer broke a bone or whether a backhoe did the damage when workers stumbled on a clandestine grave at a construction site. Through long experience, forensic practitioners learn to discern whether the trauma was premortem (before death), postmortem (after death), or perimortem (around the same time as death).

The meeting of earth and bone also leaves marks. Bones can be dyed the colors of the clothes they were buried in. Bullets, coins, and rings can leave green stains. Fungus and mold can turn bones pink, and minerals can leave them bright blue and black. Acidic soil can erode their surface. Roots can etch bones with lacy patterns and grow through skeletons, causing cracks and breaks. Dogs, rodents, and termites gnaw bones. Attracted to the decomposing corpse, beetles and wasps bore and tunnel into the skeleton. Damage, disease, and trauma can look alike. As I learn to read bones, I discover that things are not always what they seem.

Stephanie and Nicole examine the girl's skull, debating. I'm relieved when they finally give up and consult the case file, which gives a succinct outline: The remains were found in skeletonized condition, the last of seventy-four bodies exhumed from a water well at a former military base. The weight of the other remains, plus the dirt and rocks that had been used to cover the bodies, placed significant pressure on the skeleton, remodeling the shape of the skull over time. "Postmortem change," Nicole writes on our practice sheet.

Around us, everyone who has been quietly observing our progress begins to talk and laugh. We are gently teased for our failure to grasp what, to experienced forensic anthropologists, was an obvious postmortem finding. For an expert, the skull required little more than a glance. We haven't exactly passed the test with flying colors. We've revealed that we are still beginners. This comes as no news to me; I've recently articulated a skeleton with the shoulder blades reversed, a mistake at once humbling and comical but also monstrous—a Frankenstein transgression against the integrity of the body under my care. But I sense the joking stings Stephanie and Nicole.

"And the canine bones?" Stephanie asks, changing the subject.

Vicente says, "That's her dog. They were always together, so we wanted them to stay together."

His answer lands in my stomach with a thud. I have lost track of the girl in the bones. The intermingled remains weren't a trick question at all. They were about something altogether different than forensic knowledge: the love of a girl for her dog. Or maybe the bones were a trick question but asking something much bigger—asking us if we had remained ethically alert as we articulated the teaching skeleton. If we had held this girl's full humanity in our hearts. Part of learning to read these signs is remembering what is not imprinted, how much about life and death bones can never show.

. . .

VICENTE TELLS US about the case. I have the feeling he's been waiting for us to finish so he can get to the story. The team excavated the well for several weeks, starting with the bodies at the surface and working their way down. After exhuming seventy-three "probable male" bodies, they were surprised to find a "probable female" skeleton at the bottom, beside the bones of a dog. They completed the profile in the lab, but there was no match in the DNA database. The story might have ended there, with the case gone cold and the body never identified, stored in a box above the lab. But, despite other work piling up, they felt compelled to try to identify the girl. It would bring her parents some peace to have her body returned and at least be able to have a funeral. So, without many scientific clues to go on, they tried to find her family.

Oral history is an integral part of forensic work and is often used to contextualize physical evidence. It can help find clandestine burial sites: The prisoner who escaped from Xolosinay led the team to graves at the army encampment. It can help identify people. When the team collects cheek swabs from family members for DNA samples, they also collect oral histories. They ask what the missing person was wearing when they were last seen, if there was anything notable about their teeth, if they had ever suffered a major injury. A story of a kid falling off a bike and breaking a leg can be a clue to the identity of a body with a long-healed tibia fracture.

Searching for clues to the identity of the girl found in the well, the team started asking around the town nearest the exhumation site. Someone recalled a girl from a neighboring village who always had her dog with her. She often visited the military base and there were rumors that she traded sex for food for her family. For a while, it seemed like she was living on the base. Then she vanished.

*　　　　　．　．　．*

MANY WOMEN AND girls disappeared onto military bases during La Violencia. In a well-known case, women from a small Q'eqchi' Maya community called Sepur Zarco were kept against their will on a military base for months.

*　　　　　．　．　．*

THE ARMY ARRIVED in Sepur Zarco in August 1982 with a list of members of a committee petitioning the state to reclaim Q'eqchi' land from wealthy landowners. The military's scorched-earth tactic unfolded as it did in many other towns. The soldiers tortured and killed the men on the list; they raped women and girls; they burned houses and crops. But in Sepur Zarco, the military singled out the wives of the men they had massacred, holding them captive or forcing them to report for regular "duty" on the local military base, where they were compelled to cook and clean and subjected to systematic sexual violence. One woman, Dominga Cuc, was murdered, along with her two young daughters, Anita and Hermelinda. The other women understood the message: Submit, or you and your children will be killed, too.

The women suffered violence and trauma at the hands of the soldiers and social ostracism in their community. One woman described the pain of people calling her "the soldiers' woman." Another woman related how a soldier told her, "No one asks about you anymore, no one cares about you. You belong to us now."

In the years after the armed conflict, the women of Sepur Zarco slowly and steadily organized a legal case. Supported by an alliance of Indigenous women's organizations and human rights groups, fifteen Q'eqchi' Maya women brought a landmark lawsuit charging military officials with crimes against humanity. When the case went to trial in 2016, the courtroom was packed. Maya women came from all over the country carrying flowers and holding signs that read WE ARE ALL SEPUR ZARCO. The Abuelas, or grandmothers—as the women of Sepur Zarco were respectfully called—wore their shawls draped over their faces. It was a sign of the stigma that clings to sexual violence. They spoke of a "thorn in the soul" that could not be removed. They used the term "muxuk," a Q'eqchi' word that means desecration and destruction. Their faces remained hidden under their shawls as they spoke, a visually powerful reminder that the wounds they described had been inflicted on thousands of other women and girls. During the armed conflict, the Guatemalan military used sexual violence as a weapon of war. Eighty-nine percent of the victims were Indigenous women and girls.

At the trial, the Guatemalan forensic team members presented evidence of atrocity. Sexual violence does not leave marks on bones, but the fifty-one bodies exhumed near Sepur Zarco testified to the massacre of the Abuelas' families and the constant threat of violence they lived under. The panel of three judges ordered the boxes of exhumed remains to be opened. Members of the forensic team removed the bones and arranged them on a table. The crowded courtroom went silent at the sight of the skeletal remains. The Abuelas silently said prayers to protect the souls of the dead. The bones showed bullet wounds and cuts from large-bladed weapons like machetes. Many were found with ropes binding their hands, feet, and necks. The team also exhumed and identified the body of Dominga Cuc, but her daughters were not recovered; only a few pieces of their clothing were found. Dominga's mother said at the trial that her granddaughters could never be properly buried by the family because "their bones had turned to dust."

• • •

DOMINGA AND HER daughters disappeared on a military base, like the girl who went everywhere with her dog—the girl whose bones rest on the table in the lab.

The forensic evidence of the bodies exhumed from the well is consistent with a massacre. The girl's skull testifies that she was shot at close range like the other seventy-three bodies found with her. But her bones don't show "thorns in the soul"—not all violence can be recorded on the forensic forms we fill out.

The team eventually tracked down the girl's family, but were turned away. The family said it was the wrong house; they didn't have a daughter. Eventually, they said they once had a daughter, but they didn't want to talk about it. They wouldn't give DNA samples to help identify the body. They didn't want her back.

Vicente told us the story of the teaching skeleton nearly ten years after the well had been exhumed, but the team's outrage about the case was still fresh.

"I can't believe they wouldn't take her back," José said. "How could they refuse their daughter's body?"

Maybe her family didn't take her back because they were

callous—there are unhappy families everywhere on earth. Maybe they had something to hide. Maybe they were afraid—victims and perpetrators still live side by side in many Guatemalan towns. Maybe it was a response to trauma, an act of self-protection to avoid prodding a painful wound. For whatever reason, the girl was, in a sense, orphaned in death.

. . .

FORENSIC EXHUMATION IS carried out in service of justice and in service of the families of the disappeared. The girl found in the well cannot be said to have been accommodated on either point. The state has not brought her murderers to justice and her family did not extend their care to her.

Julia tells me, "We keep her here with us. We want her. She is one of us." And so, the girl and her dog stay in the lab. She isn't kept in the lab solely to be a teaching skeleton; she is kept to give her story a different ending—one in which she is claimed and wanted.

She has taught a generation of forensic practitioners about gunshot trauma and postmortem changes to the skull. She also teaches what is not written on bone. Year after year, groups of students puzzle over her skeleton, sorting out human and canine bones. Her body is pieced together over and over. Her profile is completed time and again. Each time her body is articulated, her story is told. Bones and story together, we catch a glimpse of her full humanity. This is not a funeral rite, but it is a ritual. This is not a proper burial, but it is a way to honor the dead. This isn't justice, but it is a form of testimony.

. . .

ON FEBRUARY 26, 2016, a Guatemalan court found the former military officials of Sepur Zarco guilty of crimes against humanity. The verdict was groundbreaking. It was the first time that a

Guatemalan court prosecuted a case of sexual violence related to the armed conflict, and the first time that such a case was tried in the country where the violence took place. Furthermore, the case affirmed the crucial role of the testimony of survivors rather than relying on physical evidence. The Abuelas' words spoke eloquently to the marks left on spirits that were no longer visible on bodies.

When the sentence was handed down, the audience in the packed courtroom erupted in cheers, chanting "Justice! Justice!" The Maya women who had come from all over the country embraced in the aisles, and the Abuelas, from beneath their shawls, lifted their hands in victory.

CHAPTER 6

The Ghosts of Argentina

I ARRIVE IN BUENOS AIRES in December. It is summer in Argentina, vacation time. I'm disoriented by the (to me) upside-down seasons of the Southern Hemisphere. The field school in Guatemala has ended, and my fieldwork in Argentina has not yet begun. I am in between things. I have come to Argentina because this is where forensic exhumation for human rights as we know it began. Forty years ago, the military dictatorship undertook a campaign of disappearance on a massive scale, kidnapping and killing up to thirty thousand people and secretly disposing of the dead. With the fragile return of democracy in 1984, a group of university students started to look for the missing. Pioneering the application of forensic and archaeological methods to investigate human rights abuses, they created the "world's first professional war crimes exhumation team." From the violence of the Argentine dictatorship, a new field was forged.

Despite this history, Buenos Aires feels carefree. Tourists drink café cortados at sidewalk tables in Recoleta, and families meander Palermo Soho at midnight eating ice cream cones. I am a world away from Guatemala City with its barred windows and cautious streets. It is hard to believe that a few weeks ago, I was standing in the mud of an excavation site. Walking through leafy Parque Centenario, I watch students in an outdoor yoga class simultaneously fold themselves into downward dog. When I stumble across sidewalk plaques called baldosas commemorating the locations where people were kidnapped (in front of an

apartment block, outside a school, next to a hospital), I am sometimes startled. In Guatemala, I never forgot about violence and
death, but here I sometimes do.

The city blooms with summer pleasures, but I mostly stay
home alone. In Guatemala, I was always with other people. We
dug together and ate lunch together. We shared rooms, clothes,
mosquito spray, water bottles, and colds. In Argentina, I am on
my own. My newly rented studio apartment is clinically bare and
white: white-tiled floor, white walls, white curtains. It's like living inside an eggshell. In this luminous box, I feel as weak and
awkward as a hatchling, with its blind and lolling oversize head.
My head, too, seems too big and unbalanced. When do I realize I
am not well? When I hear people laughing as they pass on the
street and rush to close the curtains? When I skip dinner and sit
hungry on the edge of my bed rather than go outside? Odd things
enter my mind: A woodcut print at my mother's house of children in a garden. Above them, puffy summer clouds. Below
them, roots of trees and plants sinking into the earth—and tan-
gled among the roots, skeletons.

I constantly think of the bones crisscrossed in the dirt, their
precise pattern. Why this grave and not one of the others? I don't
know, but the exhumation with the three men is always there,
like a radio playing in the background. The strata of copper-
tinged soil. The women from the community, arms folded, waiting at the edge of the excavation. The smell of earth. The bones.
I think of them all the time, but especially at night, lying awake,
listening to the hum of the air conditioner pumping out a luke-
warm breeze.

The trick for getting through the night is to cut it down to size.
Make it as brief as possible. It was easier in Guatemala. The
fieldwork days in El Quiché had martial precision. We met for
breakfast at 6:00 A.M., crowded around long, plastic-covered tables with our plates of scrambled eggs and tortillas. By 6:30, we'd

divided into groups and piled into pickups heading to exhumation sites or rural communities to collect DNA samples from
families of the disappeared. At the exhumation site, women from
the local community prepared us pots of rice and stew for lunch
at noon. By 4:00, we started closing the site for the day to make
the long drive back to town. We met for dinner at the same place
we had breakfast, hanging around the table afterward to chat or
play cards. Then we retreated to our rooms. This was a dangerous time. In the field, my room was a cement box with a bunker
window bolted shut. It smelled like mildew and bleach. I wrote
my field notes, which were always incomplete. I would need
twelve hours to write about a twelve-hour day, like the Jorge
Luis Borges story in which the map of the Empire grew to the
size of the Empire. I closed my computer and switched off the
bulb dangling from the ceiling. If I was lucky, day and night
formed an immediate seal. I was often lucky because, as Don
Jaime observed, I was not used to physical labor, and I was always exhausted.

In these nights in Buenos Aires, I am usually not lucky, and a
blade of anxiety inserts itself between day and night, prying
them apart like an oyster. I lie awake with the bones, the graves,
and the stories of horror hovering in the dark.

.   .   .

ONE HOT AFTERNOON, someone knocks on the white door of my
white apartment. I answer reluctantly. A woman smiles and introduces herself. She lives upstairs. She is from Colombia, here
to study dentistry. She tells me that Colombian students rent
half the apartments in the building. The nearly sixty-year armed
conflict in their country is amorphous and ongoing, sparked by a
decade of conflict known as "La Violencia," the violence, the
term also used in Guatemala. As in Guatemala, mass graves dot
the map of Colombia. Argentina has always been a country of

immigrants, attracting refugees and migrants from across Latin America and around the world. Many newcomers end up in villas miserias, literally "misery towns," hard-knock favelas scattered across the city. Others, like my neighbor, land on their feet in comfortable apartment buildings pursuing professional degrees. She has come to invite me to a barbecue. "You can't spend Christmas alone!" She smiles. There is a smudge of lipstick on her perfect white teeth.

. . .

TOOTHBRUSHES, BROOMS, DUSTPANS, pink and green plastic buckets. On the way to the exhumation site, Maxi stops at the Walmart on the outskirts of Guatemala City to buy supplies. The tools for excavating mass graves are ordinary. We work for hours cleaning dirt off the three bodies, careful not to displace their position in the grave. Brushing away the dirt with a toothbrush, we find a cord still tied around the intricate carpal bones of one man's wrists. His shirt is intact and colorful. The stitching is even and sewn by hand. Some of the thread along the sleeve has rotted away (cotton degrades faster than nylon), and the unstitched fabric has reverted to pattern pieces. I imagine his wife or mother cutting and sewing the cloth. His ribs are sharp beneath the material.

Maxi tells me that when bodies are found wearing traje, traditional clothing, women from the community often ask for photographs of the huipil and sometimes climb into the grave to inspect the embroidery of the blouse. Each handwoven huipil is unique and can give a clue to the identity of the bones. If a woman finds her mother's body, she may have the exact huipil made for herself and her daughters.

Recognition by huipil is not scientific identification. Bodies are sometimes found with distinctive jewelry, unusual tattoos, and even identification documents. Such evidence is recorded and can help establish identity, dependent on the findings of forensic analysis and, ideally, a DNA match. But ID cards can end up with someone other than their original owner. People have similar tattoos. Jewelry gets stolen. Clothes get switched.

Yet families may find clothing more convincing than a forensic identification or even a DNA match. It can be hard to recognize a son or a mother in a skeleton—or a fragment of bone, or a genetic analysis with its string of numbers and probability percentage. A watch, a ring, a driver's license, a huipil—any familiar object may feel far more powerfully linked to the missing person. Families and forensic teams may find certainty in different forms of proof.

In Guatemala, dreams offer essential evidence. In the Maya Cosmovision, the living and the dead maintain a vital relationship, and dreams are the primary means by which the dead communicate.

The dead remain part of life—they aren't even precisely dead. An Achí Maya man from the village of Rabinal explained to a researcher: "They live, they're not dead. They're more alive than we are." The dead continue to work, love, and worry. Everyday objects must be buried in the grave because the dead will use them for what comes next. Like the living, the dead have needs and require care.

When the dead are not properly buried, they can become restless and upset; they "lloran y gritan," cry and scream. Proper burial is not simply a matter of respect but of urgency to ensure that the dead are at peace, the living flourish, and the relationship between them is harmonious. The ancestors are part of the community, and if they are well cared for, they will be protectors and guides. The living care for the dead so that the dead will care for the living.

All societies care for their dead and perform mourning rites. But societies have different understandings of how death rituals benefit the living and the dead. In contemporary North American funerals, we say that the dead should "rest in peace," but our emphasis is on the welfare of the grieving family. When a body cannot be properly buried, for example, after the 9/11 attacks, our primary cultural concern centers on how the absence of the body affects the grief process of the mourners. In Guatemala, the emphasis is on the well-being of the dead.

La Violencia devastated the living, but its pain also reverberates through the dead, who cry and scream, who are restless and need care so that they can take their rightful place in relation to the world of the living. Unsettled spirits can bring misfortune. Sites of massacres and areas near clandestine graves are considered dangerous places, known for fatal car crashes, deadly falls, and other accidents. The dead can communicate through sickness, like headaches, pain, and fever. Some people attributed a measles epidemic in 1990 to the ill effects of so many unburied dead. But the primary way that the dead make their discontent known is through dreams.

Dreams are important in Maya communities. In traditional practice, partners wake each other up at night to discuss and analyze them, and children are encouraged to share their dreams each morning. Because La Violencia brought staggering death, it also brought survivors dreams of the dead.

When exhumations began in the early 1990s, the dead appeared in dreams, telling their family members where their bodies were buried, instructing them where to look for mass graves.

"They start talking in dreams," explains Rosalina Tuyuc, a Kaqchikel Maya human rights leader whose father and husband were disappeared in La Violencia. "They even begin to guide our work to say, 'Well, I won't be in such a place, they won't find me.' Or 'I will be in such a tree. I am waiting for you.'" In a story related by the Guatemalan forensic team, a woman named Isabel was searching for her son and her father-in-law, but two attempts at exhumation were unsuccessful. One night, her father-in-law, Don Sebastián, appeared to Isabel in a dream and told her not to give up, that they were "just a little further up." Their bodies were exhumed a few meters from where the forensic team had been working, as the dream predicted.

During an exhumation in a cave, a woman visited daily, looking for her son. She thought that one of the bodies uncovered might be her boy, but she was distressed because she couldn't remember what he was wearing the day he disappeared, and she wasn't sure it was him. Then she had a dream that her son was in a house with many doors, dressed in the clothes she had seen in the grave. He said, "Thank you, Mom, now I am free," and left. She tried to follow him but couldn't and woke up.

Kaqchikel Maya psychologist Mónica Esmeralda Pinzón González interviewed a woman who had a dream about her missing husband the night before an exhumation. He appeared in old-fashioned clothing of coarse cotton and took off his hat, using it to show her where he was buried—near a ditch with white stones. The following day the exhumation began, but after hours of work digging trenches in a hillside, no bodies were found. The woman shared her dream, and soon her husband's body was discovered in a ditch, just as he'd said it would be.

Community members find evidence for locating graves in dreams, but forensic teams are trained to find archaeological indications. They look for subtle changes in the topography like sunken areas, and examine the soil, searching for signs in its color and texture that it has been disturbed. I once asked Zulma about these different approaches. She diplomatically told me that the Maya Cosmovision and scientific practices are both valid and must be respected. She said that technologies like genetic testing are important for Maya communities, and so are dreams. When I asked if she feels like the forensic team takes the dreams reported to them seriously, she said that they do, adding, "But we have to be patient with the scientists. They have a different way of seeing the world." She says, "More than anything, they are interested in the color of soil, but we are more interested in dreams."

I talked to Alvaro, who said community members often report dreams indicating where to search for bodies. Just that week, a woman had approached him to relate a dream that her father was buried at the current site "under a big pine tree." I asked if the team would search there, and he said they would try. "We have to respect the way they see the world," he said, echoing Zulma's phrase. Then he sighed and said, "But there are a lot of pine trees!"

There are many dead buried beneath the trees of Guatemala. In the three decades of searching for the missing, the forensic team and Maya communities have worked to find common ground, to balance science and the sacred, and to pay careful attention to mixed earth and dreams. Teams and families have learned to see the same tree in more than one way. Zulma told me that sometimes it can be tricky to navigate, but with patience and wisdom, they manage it. She explained that even if you don't believe the bones have a soul or spirit, even if you think that "a bone can be thrown anywhere or broken and feel nothing," you will still accept that every victim deserves a dignified burial. You will still understand that no one should be left in a mass grave. "If they were left in a forest, if they were left at the edge of a river, if they were left by the side of a road, wherever they were left, they did not choose that place; they did not want to be there." So the evidence you find most compelling matters less than the shared goal of finding the victims of La Violencia. Zulma said everyone is working to properly bury the dead in a cemetery, where they can rest in peace and their families can visit them on the Day of the Dead.

Zulma's sister was disappeared during the height of La Violencia. Her body has not been found, though Zulma searches tirelessly. She has appeared to Zulma in dreams to tell her that she is lying near a river. She says that she is cold. "That is why we must find her."

• • •

IN MY WHITE apartment in Argentina, I read academic articles and books on exhumations in Spain, Cyprus, and Rwanda, but I can't concentrate. Instead of printed text, I see the tidy bullet holes in two of the crania. The third is completely shattered. A scapula is marked with lines that I've learned are from machete blows. The telltale cuts are found on many bones, including femurs, tibias, and low on the fibula because, with a severed Achilles tendon, people can't run away.

• • •

IN GUATEMALA, WE are digging near a large pine tree, whose roots make the shoveling hard going. It is already late in the day when we find the first bone. The air is heavy with approaching rain. As Alvaro scrapes away the earth from the femur, the local men prepare a tarp to protect the site from the impending storm. In a flash of a machete blade, they chop branches from trees, cutting supports and cleverly notching stakes to fit together, making tents over the open pits in minutes. Maxi once said that one of the tragedies of La Violencia was that it disgraced the machete. It brought shame to a noble instrument that harvests maize and builds houses. So much suffering dealt by machetes, so many massacres. A tool of life made a weapon of death.

• • •

IN THE ARGENTINE summer, I look at the hands of men I pass on the street, men who make change for me in shops, men reading newspapers on the subway. I imagine the hands of strangers holding machetes. In Argentina, cattle prods were the weapon of choice for torture. For killing, the military favored guns and pushing prisoners from planes, drugged but alive, into the ocean or the wide brown Río de la Plata.

"Genocide" is a misleading word. Its violence dressed up in Greek and Latin, it sounds like "pesticide," like something sprayed from a bottle at arm's length. But violence is often intimate, taking place body to body. A man ties a ligature or a blindfold with the same dexterous movements that the guy at the corner vegetable stand knots my bag of tomatoes. A trigger is squeezed between thumb and forefinger in the same motion that a coin is picked up from the floor. A fist closes around a machete, a hand grabs a newborn's tender ankle, two palms rest against a young man's back.

In *Precarious Life*, philosopher Judith Butler argues for an ethics founded on our shared human condition as vulnerable bodies. She writes: "The body implies mortality, vulnerability, agency: the skin and the flesh expose us to the gaze of others, but also to touch, and to violence." It is also with the body that we gaze at others, caress them, and hurt them. Vulnerability is the basis of care and harm, compassion and torture.

Hands are menacing. Violence feels as possible and ordinary as handshaking, backslapping, or lighting a cigarette. It seems possible that the grocer, the man sitting next to me on the bus, or the man holding his daughter's hand as they cross the street could have severed a prisoner's Achilles or smashed the soft skull of a baby. If they have not, it seems less like innocence than an accident of history.

Something dark seeps into the carefree days of the Buenos Aires summer. The baldosas in front of the ordinary places where people were disappeared no longer surprise; they announce *it can happen anywhere*.

• • •

THE LANDLORD FIXES the air conditioner, but I can't sleep. I try to keep the thoughts of death at bay by thinking about life. About the people I love. About the beauty stored in the future. About falling in love and having a child. But, lying awake at night, I ask myself how it is possible to stand in a mass grave and still want to bring a child into this broken world. In this world, soldiers break the heads of children against trees, melon-split. In this world, Vicente tells me about unwrapping a woman's body, unwinding the material, peeling back the fabric, and finding in the last layer the tiny bones of the infant on her back.

• • •

IN GUATEMALA, THE rain begins to pour down, but we keep working under the tarp, fueled by excitement that we have found a grave. Within an hour, the distinct forms of three skeletonized bodies are visible. On the ride back to town, as the truck inches through the downpour, Maxi and Alvaro tell a story. During an exhumation in another community, a hard rain began to fall. The excavated pit with its half-exposed bodies quickly filled with water. Community members jumped in to pull out the bones, to save the people buried there from drowning. The punch line of this story is, of course, that the dead can't drown. Yet, with our pickaxes and DNA tests, we, too, are always trying to save them.

A story about drowning the dead marks a boundary between the team and the families. It separates a scientific conception of the corpse from an understanding of the dead as still in some sense vital—the dead who lloran y gritan. The line between science and the sacred might seem unassailable, but I feel less and less sure about the stability of such divisions. Take dreams. Like community members, people on forensic teams also dream of the dead. Alvaro says, "This work gives us all bad dreams. Re-

petitive dreams." He says that after three months at an exhumation site, "the team is haunted." He tells me, "We have to distance
ourselves—not dehumanize, but distance."

"Can you do that?" I ask.

"Yes," he says and turns away, ending the conversation.

In the early years of the Guatemalan team's work, director
Fredy Peccerelli was excavating a mass grave at a cardamom
drying plant where four hundred people had been massacred.
The team was staying in tents at the site. Local people stopped by
and described how soldiers had killed children by swinging their
heads against a support post, pointing to a beam near where
Fredy had set up camp. After that, he dreamed that he was sleeping in pools of blood. Mimi Doretti, a founding member of the
Argentine forensic team, dreamed that a skeleton emerged from
a closet dressed in her sister's clothes. Other team members
have dreamed of dismembered legs in their beds, swimming
pools filled with severed torsos, and digging up a brother's body.
I dream that bones are arranged under my bed and that I must
lie still to protect them, hide them, and keep them safe. I dream
of looking down at my body and seeing that I am a skeleton and
feeling surprised. It happened so fast.

Maxi contradicts these accounts. He says, "No one dreams.
You stop dreaming after the first few months." He tells me he
hasn't had a dream in years. Whether dreams effloresce or
wither, they seem to mark dangerous territory.

A joke circulates on forensic teams: *My therapist is Doctor
Jameson,* referring to a bottle of whiskey. A few nights of drinking punctuate the exhumation. Gallo beer and Quetzalteca liquor (no one can afford Jameson) loosen tongues. Gossip flows
and friends are teased. Occasionally, things take a darker turn.
In the anecdotes shared, I sometimes hear the dead *lloran y gritan.*

The line between the scientific and sacred treatment of the

dead wavers. The boundary sometimes seems more like a porous membrane than a cement wall. In an interview with a journalist, an Argentine forensic team member remarked that she abhors the part of the lab protocol that requires her to place skulls in plastic bags: "It's stupid but I feel like they're suffocating." Some forensic team members say that sawing bones for DNA sampling or crushing them for analysis disturbs them. These are not strictly scientific reactions. The worry of suffocation is not so different from the worry of drowning.

Perhaps the boundaries between science and sacred don't divide teams from families but enclose them in the same field—the common ground of caring for the dead. The field of care includes studying the color of the soil and examining the stitching of a huipil. It encompasses dreams and DNA. As Zulma said, everyone is trying to bury the dead properly.

As far back as we can trace human societies, the dead body has never been meaningless matter; the corpse has always been treated with ritual. Caring for the dead is a primordial human act—a mark of humanness as essential as language or tool use. Families and forensic teams share this human duty. It is the job of the living to save the dead from drowning.

. . .

THE GHOSTS ARRIVE on a bright, hot afternoon. I am in my white apartment, sitting cross-legged on my white bed, listening to a guided meditation on YouTube. I am trying to feel better. I breathe in and out. Bullet holes in skulls. I breathe in. Cut marks of machete on bone. I breathe out. The dead. The graves. In Guatemala. In Argentina. Colombia, Bosnia and Herzegovina, Cambodia, Cyprus, Rwanda, Spain, Sri Lanka, Ukraine, Zimbabwe. You could go through the alphabet, stick pins in a map. Mass graves pockmark the globe. Terrible things have happened, and terrible things are happening now. The entire world is slick and sticky with blood. Breathe in and out.

I turn off my meditation and decide to take a shower to wash away these thoughts. It is as if I'm suffering from some strange form of synesthesia, but instead of colors turning into sounds or shapes becoming tastes, everything transforms into the grave. Things only get worse under the water. I am drowning in images of horror. Toweling my hair, I walk back into the white room. They are standing there, milling in front of the kitchen sink. They are lively flesh, not skeletons, and there are no marks of violence on them. There are three of them. But one is a woman. The two men wear work clothes and rubber boots, but she wears traje; her simple huipil is white, with just a little embroidery. I wonder how we missed that one of the bodies was female. She must have been dressed in men's clothes. Or maybe she was the body below the other two, the one that we did not manage to fully expose before I left the site. They look tired from traveling so far, and they are dirty from the grave. Their posture is tentative, almost apologetic, and I realize it is because they feel bad about the muddy footprints they have tracked on the white floor. One of the men speaks to me briefly, with kindness and concern. Then they are gone. I stand in the white room alone, naked.

• • •

THE VISITATION WAS most comparable to a dream. While it unfolded, I was immersed in it. When it was over, it vanished. It was not unreal or imaginary; it simply belonged to another category of existence, as waking and sleeping are different states of being. It was like the optical illusion in which you look one way and see a vase and look another and see a woman's profile, but you can never see both at once. Look this way, and the ghosts are real. Look this way, and you have some sort of PTSD.

Optical illusions like the "Rubin vase" invoke a phenomenon called "multistable perception." Struggling to make sense of ambiguous information, our visual systems decode an image one way, then another, in what are known as "perceptual reversals." We are wired to make sense of things, and when things are too uncertain and complex to interpret, we oscillate between possible explanations, unable to settle on one.

Catastrophic violence overwhelms sense-making. How can people inflict such suffering on one another? How much grief is in a mass grave? Atrocity invokes a form of multistable perception; unable to assimilate the magnitude of horror, the mind reels between different systems of meaning. The ritual and the analytical buzz in electric proximity. Science and ghosts, blue on red, snap in and out of focus. There is no stable place to land when confronting the world's violence.

In the perceptual reversals of fieldwork, from one perspective, I worked with forensic teams to care for the dead. From another, the dead appeared to care for me. Only the first state sustains analysis, supports a dissertation, and offers itself to academia. The other is a shadow. I did not tell anyone about the ghosts. Who would I tell? My mother and worry her? My PhD adviser and fail the ritual of fieldwork? Or worse, become an object of study? I did a literature review; I found that experiences of visual and auditory hallucination are relatively common, not necessarily pathological. I copied the citations into a document in Chicago style. I kept it to myself. Perhaps I sensed that any response would be wrong: Some people would speak to the profile and some to the vase, but never to both together, never to address the strange tension between them.

That evening, I cleaned my apartment. I washed the white-tiled floors. Wringing out the mop, I was confused that the water ran clear when it should have been muddy from the boot tracks of the visitors from Guatemala.

The ghosts appeared. They vanished. I was neither healed nor harmed. I continued to be haunted by what I had seen in the graves of Guatemala and what was waiting for me in the graves of Argentina. I never found the right distance like Alvaro advised or stopped dreaming like Maxi. I never settled on the profile or the vase. Yet I was comforted by the ghosts' visit. It helped me go on.

•   •   •

THE WEEK AFTER the ghosts appeared, I wrote to Maxi to ask about the grave in the hills of El Quiché. He wrote back to say it was bigger than they thought. Sixteen bodies so far. He didn't mention if there were any probable female remains recovered. He said they found more bodies deeper down, as expected, but also slightly to the south, under the pine tree.

CHAPTER 7

Tucumán Is Burning

G RIPPING MY TICKET and bag, I run through Retiro station. The screens listing departures aren't working, and the public announcements are too crackly to understand. Faded travel posters for Iguazú Falls and Perito Moreno Glacier line the corridors. There is a saying that "Buenos Aires isn't Argentina," and bus trips teach me how vast the country is and how varied its landscapes. About a third of the population are porteños, residents of Buenos Aires, and the rest are scattered around a territory five times the size of France. Under the dictatorship, the grid of military control extended across the country, from the tropical province of Misiones bordering Brazil to the ice fields of Patagonia.

I find my bus just in time, and an employee with a clipboard ushers me aboard the double-decker for the eighteen-hour trip north. As the bus speeds through the vast pampas in the dark, I read *A Lexicon of Terror,* a celebrated book about how the dictatorship deformed and twisted language, turning ordinary words into codes for violence. The author, Marguerite Feitlowitz, asked those who had lived through the years of repression, "What words can you no longer tolerate? What words do you no longer say?" The first entry in her lexicon is "desaparecido/a (noun)." Someone who has been disappeared. "The first thing they told me was to forget who I was, that as of that moment I would be known only by a number, and that for me the outside world stopped there."

I have been compiling my own lexicon of horror in Argentina. Stories of the dictatorship have changed how I see ordinary things. Green cars, metal bed frames, sugar factories, and hot chocolate have been imprinted with new meanings.

．．．

THE MILITARY SEIZED control of Argentina on March 24, 1976. Flanked by Catholic bishops, General Jorge Rafael Videla, Admiral Emilio Eduardo Massera, and Brigadier General Orlando Ramón Agosti appeared on television to deliver earnest speeches about faith, family, and the fatherland. Videla was the first to serve as de facto president. From a military family, Videla attended the Colegio Militar de la Nación and the Escuela Superior de Guerra. He later taught military intelligence, served as part of Argentina's mission to the Inter-American Defense Board in Washington, D.C., and trained in counterinsurgency at the School of the Americas. With his slight build and dapper mustache, dressed in Scottish tweeds and pocket squares when not in uniform, he seemed more like a high school principal than a tyrant. In early interviews with the press, Videla gave soft-spoken and detailed answers to reporters' queries. Neither bombastic nor threatening, he sounded reasonable, even dull. Yet the "licensed sadism" of the dictatorship's seven-year rule was already underway.

The junta immediately introduced El Proceso de Reorganización Nacional (Process for National Reorganization), a plan to restructure the country politically, economically, and socially—but also spiritually. Its aim, as described by General Videla, was to bring about a "profound transformation of consciousness." "El Proceso," as it was commonly called, is also the Spanish title of Kafka's novel *The Trial*, which tells the story of a man's inexplicable arrest and assassination for an unknowable crime by an all-powerful state—perhaps an early clue to the hallucinatory quality of the junta's violent rule. A dizzying gap grew between appearance and reality, between certain knowledge and what Hannah Arendt calls the "common sense disinclination to believe the monstrous," between Videla's tweedy speeches that called for "the energetic protection of human rights" and the blood on the general's hands. As Arendt observes, "The ideal subject of totalitarian rule is not the convinced Nazi or the convinced Communist, but people for whom the distinction between fact and fiction (i.e., the reality of experience) and the distinction between the true and the false (i.e., the standards of thought) no longer exist."

The junta commanded death squads but also the opera and popular magazines. There were secret prisons and public festivities. At Videla's behest, New York public relations firm Burson-Marsteller ran a twelve-page supplement in *The New York Times Magazine* celebrating Argentina's "untold natural riches" and "vivacious, adaptable people" in a bid to improve the country's image. In 1978, Argentina hosted the World Cup. While fans from around the world celebrated the Argentine team's victory in the streets, people being held in clandestine detention centers could hear the cheering crowds from their torture chambers.

chupadero (noun), from the Spanish verb chupar, to suck. A clandestine detention center where people are sucked up and never seen again.

chupado/a (noun), the person who has been sucked up, i.e., the prisoner.

tratamiento (noun), literally "treatment," meaning torture.

vuelo (noun), "flight," the practice of throwing sedated prisoners to their deaths from airplanes.

The entries for disappearance, torture, and death in *A Lexicon of Terror* follow closely.

By the time the junta issued their first decrees and filled the radio waves with military marches, Argentina had been reeling between dictatorship and democracy for nearly fifty years.

The key figure in twentieth-century Argentine politics was Juan Domingo Perón, who served three terms as president, winning his first election in 1946 and his last in 1973. He dominated Argentine politics for three decades and still does: Elections in the twenty-first century are battles between Perónist and anti-Perónist candidates.

Perón rose to power with the support of the working class, who embraced his "third way" between capitalism and communism. Under Perón, women got the vote, real wages increased, and the standard of living for ordinary people improved dramatically. Perón implemented progressive social reforms, expanding access to healthcare and education. He nationalized the largely British-owned railways and paid off Argentina's foreign debt. His first presidency was a time of prosperity and optimism, a "chain effect of happiness." Workers had money in their pockets and a sense of dignity. For the first time, many had paid vacations and flocked to the seaside resort of Mar del Plata, which saw a three-fold increase in visitors between 1940 and 1955. Perón's populist government gained a devoted following, bolstered by his charismatic wife, María Eva Duarte de Perón, affectionately known as Evita. Through the Eva Perón Foundation, she founded orphanages, distributed Christmas presents to the poor, and personally answered thousands of letters and requests for help. With her Hollywood blond hair and red lipstick, her humble origins, and her skills as an orator honed on radio soap operas, she had an intense connection with Perón supporters, whom she called "mis descamisados," my shirtless ones. They called her the Lady of

Hope, the Good Fairy, the Martyr of Labor, the Standard Bearer of the Humble, and Santa Evita.

In 1952, at the height of her popularity and power, Evita died of cancer; she was thirty-three years old. In the years after her death, Perón's government moved toward totalitarianism with increasing demands for party loyalty. His relationship with the Catholic Church soured and his ties with the army, once strong, began to fray. In 1955, the military overthrew the weakened president. From exile in Spain, Juan Perón still tried to exercise political influence while Argentina careened between military and civilian governments.

• • •

In May 1969, a massive uprising against dictator Juan Carlos Onganía broke out in the city of Córdoba. Protesters took to the streets, united by shared resentment of a government that forbade everything from labor strikes to miniskirts. Working-class unionists and university students barricaded avenues; Marxists marched with leftist priests. The protests were crushed, leaving twelve dead and ninety-three wounded by official counts, and likely many more. "El Cordobazo" had unleashed popular discontent that could not be put back in a bottle. It vitalized and radicalized the left—and it mobilized a guerrilla movement.

When the dust settled, two important militant factions emerged. The largest, the Montoneros, were leftist Perónists agitating for his return to power and supported by a sizable, unarmed youth movement, the Juventud Perónista. The Ejército Revolucionario del Pueblo (People's Revolutionary Army, or ERP), was smaller and inspired by the Cuban revolution and native son Ernesto Guevara. Originally from the Argentine city of Rosario, "Che" had earned his famous nickname while working as a doctor in Guatemala, where he witnessed the U.S.-backed overthrow of Jacobo Árbenz Guzmán, an event that deepened his militancy.

The ERP believed in Guevara's "foco" theory that a small group of guerrillas in an out-of-the-way place could start a Cuban-style revolution. They gathered armed fighters in the hills of Tucumán. The northern province's long history of poverty and strong union base made it an ideal place to light a revolutionary spark. Soon, the area was a hotbed of guerrilla activity. In those years, there was a phrase for the fervor: "Tucumán arde"—Tucumán is burning.

. . .

MY BUS PULLS into the station in San Miguel de Tucumán in the late afternoon. Cars grid the once-grand avenues, and dusty orange trees line the streets. Tucumán was settled at the edge of the Inca Empire, its name coming from either the Quechua word for "the place where rivers meet" or perhaps the word "tucma," which means "the end of things." It feels like the last traces of an old Argentina, its history haphazardly preserved in the central palm-shaded squares and majestic public buildings, which give way to neighborhoods of concrete apartment blocks, and finally to shacks on the outskirts of town. Railroad tracks, built by the British to ship the white gold of sugar, stitch the fields to the city.

. . .

IN THE EARLY days, the Montoneros and ERP won popular support by carrying out daring "Robin Hood" escapades like stealing grocery trucks and delivering food—and in one case, pallets of soda—to villas miserias. But their tactics could also be brutal. To fund themselves, the guerrillas kidnapped wealthy businessmen and held them for ransom. In 1970, in an act that "marked the guerrilla organizations' official birth in public life," Montoneros

abducted and executed former president General Pedro Eugenio
Aramburu, who had been a crucial figure in the military coup
that ousted Perón.

As the political situation became increasingly volatile, the exiled Perón's influence grew. Many Argentines were nostalgic for
the relative order and prosperity the country had known under
his rule with Evita. From Spain, Perón cultivated a political
image with broad appeal. His traditional union and working-
class base supported him, but he also wooed the young militant
left, peppering his speeches with references to Che and Mao Ze-
dong. Aging unionists, high school students, and armed guerrillas pinned their hopes on Perón. While he remained in Spain, he
could be all things to all people. But everything changed when he
returned to Argentina.

After eighteen years in exile, Perón arrived in Buenos Aires on
June 20, 1973. Celebrating his homecoming, more than three
million people came to greet his flight at Ezeiza Airport. Crowds
walked along the highway and waded through the Matanza
River. But as the throng approached the airport, snipers from
right-wing Perónist factions fired at left-wing Montoneros, and a
deadly gun battle broke out. Hundreds in the crowd were in-
jured, and at least a dozen people were killed, likely more—there
was never an official investigation of the events. The dream of an
Argentina united under Perón was over before his flight touched
down on the tarmac.

. . .

IN TUCUMÁN, I meet Valeria. She tells me about going to Ezeiza
to greet Perón's flight. She walked all night with Dario, her
compañero—an ambiguous word that can mean colleague, com-
rade, or lover. They were already active Montoneros and were
sure that Perón would bring about the socialist change they'd
been fighting for. When the gunfire broke out, Dario grabbed

her hand. "That's when I knew he loved me," she says. In this middle-aged woman, with a job in public administration and practical shoes, I see the young revolutionary in love.

Valeria and I are sitting in an old-fashioned café. We order medialunas from a menu that probably hasn't changed in fifty years, except, of course, for the prices, constantly adjusted to keep pace with the frantic fluctuations of the peso. Among the Argentine classics like empanadas, tea sandwiches, and banana milkshakes, there is a "submarino"—a chocolate bar served to be melted in warm milk, a childhood treat.

> submarino (noun), a common form of torture in
> clandestine detention centers during the dictatorship.
> A method of waterboarding prisoners with feces-
> contaminated water.

The horrors of the junta are printed in the text of everyday life. Valeria tears open a pack of sugar and stirs it into her coffee. Several of the secret torture centers in Tucumán were in old sugar mills: La Nueva Baviera, Lules, Bella Vista. When our cups are empty, it is time for Valeria to go. She needs to pick up her daughter from work. Valeria was pregnant when Dario was disappeared. Their daughter knows her father only from old photos and stories like the one about the Ezeiza massacre. We say goodbye. Pushing back her chair, Valeria brushes the medialuna crumbs off her shirt, gathers her bag, and walks out of the café in her comfortable shoes, in the everyday victory of survival.

. . .

AFTER THE EZEIZA massacre, Perón embraced his right-wing supporters and disavowed the Montoneros, saying that "Marxists, subversives, and terrorists" had "infiltrated" the party. Surprisingly, the Montoneros did not abandon Perón. Instead, they blamed his treachery on his inner circle. They pointed to the Rasputin-like influence of the minister of social welfare, José López Rega, known as "El Brujo," the sorcerer, because of his reputation for dabbling in black magic. They blamed Perón's third wife and eventual vice president, Isabel Martínez de Perón, known as Isabelita, whom they hated with a ferocity inversely proportionate to their adoration of Evita. The Montoneros adopted the slogan "If Evita were alive, she would be a Montonero," and published an underground magazine called *Evita Montonera*.

Juan Perón, whose health had been faltering even before his return to Argentina, died in July 1974. Isabelita inherited the presidency. She was the first woman in the world to serve in the role of president, but she was ill-equipped to lead a nation in crisis. Lacking Evita's political instincts and charisma, she leaned heavily on El Brujo, whose shadowy presence imbued her government with sinister magic. This was not Evita's enchantment. It did not make Isabelita a beacon of hope but a political black hole, despised by the left and right alike. She alienated even Perón's most ardent supporters: Her presidency saw the first-ever union strike against a Perónist government. She was once greeted by a crowd of fifty thousand people chanting, "There is only one Evita!" For its part, the right depicted her as "hysterical and out-of-control"; before the coup, General Videla publicly spoke of the "visibly deteriorated" office of the presidency under Isabelita.

El Brujo organized a notorious secret death squad, the Alianza Anticomunista Argentina—the Triple A—which he directed from his offices in the Ministry of Social Welfare. He first unleashed the Triple A against journalists, artists, and academics. In February 1975, Isabelita's government directly targeted the guerrillas in "Operation Independence," which empowered the military to use any means necessary "to neutralize and/or annihilate the activities of subversive elements in Tucumán province." With this decree, the already weakened ERP was defeated. If Tucumán briefly burned with revolutionary fire, it was a flame quickly extinguished. Having vanquished the armed guerrillas, the military continued its campaign of disappearance, torture, and death, targeting an ever-widening circle of those deemed "subversive." Tucumán became a "testing ground for developing genocidal social practices that would later be unleashed on society at large," in the words of Argentine sociologist Daniel Feierstein. Under Isabelita, the police and military refined the tactics that would seamlessly transition to the dictatorship. Even before the coup d'état of March 24, 1976, the genocide had begun.

. . .

I TAKE THE local bus to the old train yards in Tafí Viejo, just outside Tucumán, to meet Aníbal. A prominent figure in local organizations of families of the disappeared, he arrives wearing a Sex Pistols T-shirt and a bandanna wrapped around his forehead. Somewhere in his forties, he is a fierce activist and a mountain of a man, but he has a tender side, too: His messages arrive studded with flower and ladybug emojis, and he likes to show photos of his kids and his dog, Buddy.

Aníbal walks me through one of the abandoned factories where the trains were built. The sheer size of the buildings and the stretch of the grounds is impressive. In the nineteenth century, the railways boomed, connecting the ports of Buenos Aires to the sugar factories in Tucumán and the cattle herds of the pampas.

Argentina was once among the wealthiest countries in the world. Buenos Aires competed with New York to attract immigrants. For many, the American Dream stretched to Tierra del Fuego. In my own family's lore, two brothers went to a port in

Italy and tossed a coin to decide who would board the ship to New York and who would take the boat to Buenos Aires. The coin flip seems fanciful, but one way or another, my great-grandfather ended up in the United States, and his brother settled in Argentina. For years, increasingly distant cousins sent one another airmail letters until they lost their common language. Fates are spun by luck: Heads or tails, another ship, and I would not have written these words. A different revolution, and Argentina's economy might be thriving still, driven by its abundant natural resources and waves of hopeful immigrants. But despite its riches, the country suffered a reversal of fortune from which it has never recovered, what economists call "the Argentine Paradox."

Mighty work took place in these train yards to industrialize a country as vast as Argentina, but now it is a ghost town of empty warehouses, broken windows, and cold smokestacks. Near the factories, there is a little company town with neat grids of brick cottages. It is all a little off, misplaced in the way of colonial things, a fantasy of a green and pleasant land that isn't suited to the bright South American sun. Yet people lived their lives in this little not-quite-English town. Aníbal's mother and father met here. I imagine them walking every morning to the factories, where Aníbal's father worked as a carpenter and was active in the union, which is probably why he was targeted.

Aníbal is restless, rolling cigarettes, prowling the grounds. By a rusty bike rack, he pulls a small photo of his father from his wallet. I have seen it before in newspaper articles on Tucumán's missing. In the grainy image, he looks at the camera, chin down, gaze up. It is a formal pose, like an ID photo, but also unguarded, as if the photographer snapped the picture a moment before he anticipated. He looks like Aníbal. On the outside wall of a factory building, two rows of brass plaques commemorate disappeared train-yard workers. Aníbal points to his father's name, Facundo.

The date of his disappearance is February 1976, a month before the military coup.

. . .

THE ROTTEN FRUIT of Isabelita's presidency was easy to pluck. Argentines greeted the dictatorship with the belief that anything was better than La Presidenta. The junta, representing the army, navy, and air force, promised to revive the economy, restore civic order, and pave the way to a lasting democracy. At first, the coup received sweeping public support. The English-language daily *Buenos Aires Herald* ran an editorial that stated: "The entire nation responded with relief. . . . This was not just another coup but a rescue operation. These are not men hungry for power, but men with a duty." Its editor, Robert Cox, would later flee the country after the paper defied censorship to publish lists of the disappeared. Argentina's most celebrated writer, Jorge Luis Borges, greeted the junta by saying, "Now we are governed by gentlemen."

. . .

THE LEXICON OF horror contains long lists of clandestine detention centers: El Olimpo, El Banco, El Campito, El Vesubio, El Infierno, El Silencio, La Casita, La Casona, La Átomica, El Motel, the Sheraton, Los Plátanos, El Reformatorio.

Torture centers were hidden in military buildings and police stations but also in schools, hospitals, factories, and auto repair shops. There were torture centers in the basement of the posh Galerías Pacífico shopping mall in Buenos Aires, a Ford factory, and a busy public hospital. Of the eight hundred clandestine centers identified, two of the largest were the Navy Mechanics School (ESMA by its Spanish acronym), in a parklike campus in Buenos Aires, and La Perla, on the outskirts of the city of Córdoba, near a slaughterhouse. The first was La Escuelita de Famaillá, established in a primary school under construction outside Tucumán. At the "Little School," a battery-operated field telephone that generated electric current when the handle was cranked became an instrument of torture. There were many tools: Electric cattle prods known as picanas. Rubber batons and sandbags for beating. Chains for hanging prisoners by the feet or arms. Bathtubs for waterboarding. Scalpels. Cigarettes. Rats.

Documenting the violence, members of the truth commission wrote, "In drawing up this report, we wondered about the best way to deal with the theme so that this chapter did not turn into merely an encyclopedia of horror. We could find no way to avoid this."

There was rote violence and sadistic innovation. At the Little School, soldiers tied red bands around the necks of prisoners marked for execution. At a neighboring camp, El Arsenal, a military witness described seeing a prisoner buried alive, with only his head left outside the pit, as his torturers watered and compacted the red earth of Tucumán around his body.

. . .

MANY OF TUCUMÁN'S disappeared ended up in Pozo de Vargas, one of the largest mass graves discovered in Latin America. This is where the remains of Aníbal's father, Facundo, and Valeria's compañero, Dario, were found.

Situated next to an abandoned train track, Pozo de Vargas was a forgotten industrial well built by English engineers in the nineteenth century to power steam trains. Who thought of that old well by the weedy tracks on the outskirts of town? Someone knew it was there and had the idea to bring truckloads of dead prisoners by night to throw their bodies into the depths. From 1975 to 1979, the military hid bodies in the well, covering the corpses with rocks and dirt.

Pozo de Vargas is about 10 feet in diameter and estimated to be about 130 feet deep. Estimated—because after more than a decade of work, the team has yet to reach the bottom.

Santiago, one of the founding members of the team excavating the site, tells me about the early days. We are sitting in a small building beside the well that houses the offices of the Tucumán Archaeology, Memory, and Identity Collective (El Colectivo de Arqueología, Memoria e Identidad de Tucumán, or CAMIT). They built these offices just like they built the structure covering the well to protect it from the elements. They constructed the fence surrounding the site and joined with families to plant the saplings that memorialize the people whose bodies have been found in the Pozo. Thirteen years ago, there was nothing here, just an untended field and rumors of a mass grave.

Families of the missing, human rights groups, and local archaeologists began meeting to discuss the whispered stories that bodies of the disappeared had been buried on the Vargas farm. Neighbors said that during the dictatorship, they had seen trucks arriving at night and found footprints and traces of blood. Someone with close ties to the military had made a drunken confession about a well. The group got a warrant to search the property. In 2002, they began the excavation, searching through fields of weeds until they found the opening to the well. It took two years of work to recover the first bone fragments, definitive proof of a clandestine grave. The first genetic identification was made in 2011.

Santiago tells me about the technical challenges of the excavation and the feats of engineering required just to begin the work. When they first uncovered the well, it was full of water. They rented a pump and spent days cutting drainage channels through the fields. As the water poured out, children from the neighborhood came to play. In the photos he shows me, the children look joyful splashing in the impromptu water park. Knowing what was waiting submerged in the Pozo, I shudder.

THE HOSTEL WHERE I'm staying in Tucumán has nineteenth-century stained-glass windows and seventies-era furnishings. Before going to Pozo de Vargas, I drink instant coffee from a mug with a vintage flower pattern that I once would have found kitschy and cute but that now seems like a material trace of an era of terror. In the breakfast room, a few other travelers are planning their days. Most tourists skip Tucumán in favor of Salta. Still, among the families visiting relatives and people traveling for work, there are a few hardy souls looking for off-the-beaten-path adventure. A British couple join my table. They tell me they are on their way to see the ruins of Quilmes. They ask me what I'm doing here. I hesitate and say I'm researching the dictatorship. They look at me blankly. Most of the tourists from Europe and North America I talk to have no idea there had ever been a dictatorship in Argentina. They just know the peso is a good deal. The British tourists start to tell me about their plan to visit the wineries of Cafayate, and I proceed to ruin their breakfast by reciting entries from the encyclopedia of horror.

> parrilla (noun), an outdoor grill. Also, a common form of torture in clandestine detention centers in which a prisoner was electrocuted while shackled to a metal bed frame.
>
> asado (noun), a barbecue, often held on Sundays with the family. Also, the practice of burning prisoners' bodies with tires to hide the smell.

I pin the tourists to their seats until their dry toast is gone and their little pots of dulce de leche are scraped clean. They scurry away as soon as they can. When they've left, I regret my tirade. I almost envy how they can travel in Argentina and see only the beauty without any horror, like the children playing in the Pozo water.

. . .

"FIRST WE WILL kill all of the subversives, then we will kill all of their collaborators, then those who sympathize with subversives, then we will kill those that remain indifferent, and finally we will kill the timid," said the governor of Buenos Aires province, describing El Proceso. There were few people whom these circles of hell didn't encompass. It was dangerous for men to grow beards because it made you look like a leftist; it was dangerous for women to wear jeans because it made you look like a feminist. It was dangerous to read Marx or even *The Little Prince*. The junta held book burnings, consigning the works of Julio Cortázar, Marcel Proust, Gabriel García Márquez, Pablo Neruda, Sigmund Freud, and Antoine de Saint-Exupéry to the flames. They declared, "Just as this fire now destroys material pernicious to our Christian way of being, so too will be destroyed the enemies of the Argentine soul."

General Videla proclaimed, "A terrorist is not only someone who plants bombs, but a person whose ideas are contrary to our Western, Christian civilization." To escape scrutiny, people buried their books, women painted their nails and wore stockings, men shaved their beards. But it was a lottery. People were disappeared because they were armed guerrillas or belonged to Perónist student groups, but also because they had rented an apartment from someone deemed "subversive," because their name was found in an address book, or because an acquaintance named them in a delirium during torture. Indigenous communities, particularly Indigenous activists, may have been specifically targeted. Jewish Argentines, who made up about 1 percent of the population at the time, represented at least 10 percent of the disappeared, partly due to their strong presence in professions targeted by El

Proceso, such as psychiatry and journalism, but also because of widespread anti-Semitism in the military. Torturers flaunted their Nazi sympathies, showing off swastika key rings and tattoos. The walls of clandestine detention centers were painted with swastikas. Jewish prisoners were singled out for particular pain and humiliation.

"How did your military superiors tell you to fight the enemy?" A journalist posed this question to a former sergeant who broke his silence about the atrocities he had seen and committed in the clandestine detention center El Campito.

"Towards total extermination. Death, blood. They said that those guys, the subversives, wanted to destroy the Family, that they wanted to impose a totalitarian government, a red plan. They also told us that subversives wanted to destroy our traditions, the national being [el ser nacional]. They wanted to destroy the Church." They told the sergeant, "The homeland is in danger."

"What was the homeland for you?"

"It meant defending our way of life, which was traditional, Catholic, Western."

A torturer explained the logic to a man held in a clandestine detention center: "He told me they knew I was not involved with terrorism or the guerrillas, but that they were going to torture me because I opposed the regime, because I hadn't understood that in Argentina there was no room for any opposition to the Process of National Reorganization."

. . .

BEFORE DESCENDING INTO Pozo de Vargas, we don hazmat suits. They come in one size, extra-large, and they billow and crinkle around us. The well is deep, and air must be pumped in. Deep wells carry risks of asphyxiation from lack of oxygen and the buildup of natural gases from decomposition. There is a monitor that will sound an alarm if the air quality drops below a certain point, but I'm not sure it is plugged in. The air is thin and sour.

We squeeze into the cage of a small yellow elevator. We slowly descend, past the support beams crisscrossing the space. A ladder is attached to the brick-lined wall—once the only means of access. As we are lowered, there is a moment of complete darkness when the light from the surface is blocked and the bright work lights at the bottom are not yet illuminated. It gives me a sense of panic. Although the elevator moves slowly, I have the feeling that I am being pitched into the deep.

The elevator stops about six feet above the excavation. We climb onto a support beam and, from there, carefully drop to the ground. Santiago and El Oso, one of the archaeologists on the team, make these acrobatics look effortless, but I struggle to get solid footing. I feel in danger of slipping off the beam and crashing onto the remains. The excavation level is littered with skeletons. Standing at the bottom of the well—or rather, the current excavation level—my main impression is of chaos. It would be hard to describe this entry in the encyclopedia of horror. Skeletons are disordered, upside down, sideways. Dumped from the surface, the bodies landed in contorted positions. The strange fallen angles and the sheer number of bones make it difficult to make anatomical sense of the scene and see what connects with what. Here is a tibia rising out of the dirt, a shoe dangling. Here is a skull. Here are ripped pieces of fabric caught on humerus and ulna, like flags.

. . .

THE WORD "GENOCIDE" was created in the aftermath of World War II to describe the mass slaughter of the Holocaust. The Genocide Convention of 1948 defines the term as an act intended to destroy a "national, ethnical, racial or religious group." Originally, "political groups" were also included in the definition but ultimately left out during diplomatic negotiations. In current usage of the term, political and social groups are increasingly recognized as targets of genocide. For example, the Khmer Rouge killed more than a quarter of Cambodia's population in what has been internationally recognized as a genocide carried out for ideological reasons, rather than targeting ethnic or religious groups. "Genocide" was used to characterize the atrocities of the Argentine dictatorship by the 1984 truth commission and later codified in human rights trials. For families of the missing and other activists, the term offers a decisive refutation of the dictatorship fiction that violence was equally perpetrated by guerrillas and the military in a two-sided "Dirty War," a term used in junta propaganda.

· · ·

TO THE ENCYCLOPEDIA of horror, add statistics. Record the percentages of "people, detained in front of witnesses, who have still not reappeared."

Detained in their own homes: 62 percent

Detained in the street: 24.6 percent

Detained at work: 7 percent

Detained in their place of study: 6 percent

The "task forces," which people called patotas, or gangs, usually arrived at night. They came in green Ford Falcons without license plates. Most dressed in civilian clothes. They didn't bother covering their faces. Sometimes they cut the electricity to the entire neighborhood before the kidnapping. They blocked traffic and fired weapons. Sometimes they threw grenades and circled in helicopters, calling attention to the abduction and to their impunity. The kidnapping was not secret. It was what happened next that was unknown. There was no record of the arrest. People were not held in official jails or prisons. People simply vanished.

"I categorically deny that there exist in Argentina any concentration camps or prisoners being held in military establishments beyond the time absolutely necessary for investigation of a person captured in an operation before they are transferred to a penal establishment," announced Videla in December 1977. Disappearance was a deliberate and systematic strategy. It served the dictatorship's purposes by creating plausible deniability and sheltering them from international sanctions.

International human rights organizations recognize disappearance as a form of torture for families and friends of the missing "because of the uncertainty they experience as to the fate of the victim and because they feel powerless to provide legal, moral, and material assistance." For the prisoners held in clandestine detention centers, disappearance was also torture. Dr. Norberto Liwsky testified that during the seventy-four days he was held in the secret prison La Brigada de San Justo, the guards would say, "You're dirt." "Nobody remembers you." "You don't exist."

. . .

THERE ARE TWELVE discernible crania in the Pozo. Identifying individual bodies in the chaos of the exhumation is daunting. All exhumations are puzzles, but the Pozo has no jigsaw pieces with precise edges. The excavation is three-dimensional, sculptural, a Rubik's Cube. I work on the body Santiago has assigned me. I squat by the skull, which I assess as belonging to a young adult male, and scrape thick mud from the bones, trying to follow the trail of his vertebrae into the dirt.

Exhumation is not just a matter of removing bodies. The position of the remains is scrutinized to understand how one body relates to another. Everything around the body—clothes, shoes, blindfolds, ligatures, pieces of plastic tape—must be analyzed. Each bone must be carefully freed from the mud and dirt and "cleaned in place"—without disturbing its position. The dirt and rocks covering the bodies are scooped into bags labeled by the quadrant of the grave from where they were removed. Before the elevator was installed, the team carried the bags up the ladder. On the surface, the bags are emptied and sifted through a series of screens, to capture any fragments of bone or scraps of fabric that might have been missed. The bones and their associated "grave contents" are shipped to the forensic lab in Buenos Aires, where they will be analyzed.

El Oso balances his prodigious frame over the delicate bones. Only two or three people can work at the same time in the small space. The excavation is painstaking and often literally painful. To avoid damaging the remains, we crouch and prop ourselves in odd poses. We work in silence. We catch a floating cumbia from a car passing on the road. *We need a radio*, says El Oso. Then silence again. I glance up to see Santiago focused on cleaning dirt from the small bones of a foot. He is progressing much more quickly than I am, of course, but it is slow going, even for his experienced hands and eyes. Suddenly, he announces that it is time to stop. We have been working for three hours. In the strange timelessness of the Pozo, it has felt like ten minutes. We gather our tools, and they hoist me back onto the support beam to climb into the elevator. Stepping out on the surface, we lower our masks to drink in the fresh air.

CHAPTER 8

Touching Bones

"**P**OBRECITO**,**" says Emilia, "poor guy," as she pats the skull on the lab table. She has already determined that it belongs to a man in his early twenties—about Emilia's age. She has counted fourteen bullet entry points in his pelvis. When Cati, an experienced forensic anthropologist and senior member of the team, visits the lab in the afternoon, she examines the unusual pattern of trauma and, whistling under her breath, says whoever killed this guy wanted to make him suffer. Death from these kinds of wounds would be painful. Maybe they targeted his pelvis as a form of humiliation. She speculates that he may have been a leader in the guerrilla movement, someone the military wanted to make an example of. In photos from the 1970s, the guerrillas look like Che Guevara, with their berets and swags of bullets. I wonder how he would feel about Emilia patting his forehead and calling him pobrecito. Would he take it as an affront to the codes of revolutionary masculinity? A further emasculation? Or, after so much suffering, would he welcome the kindness of her touch?

The lab of the Argentine forensic anthropology team, Equipo Argentino de Antropología Forense (EAAF), is on the main thoroughfare in the gritty commercial zone of Once in Buenos Aires. Nearby streets are ordered by type of merchandise. Blocks of fabric shops sit next to blocks selling mannequins; blocks of cellphones lead to blocks of party supplies, everything with its kind. In this Noah's ark of wholesale and retail, the EAAF is singular.

The offices occupy two identical apartments on the second

and third floors of a once-grand building. Connected by a hall with a sweeping staircase and a birdcage elevator, the flats are matching labyrinths of rooms with tables, desks, whiteboards, and boxes of bones in storage. Posters peel from the walls, and houseplants thrive on the windowsills. Bookshelves are stacked with forensic textbooks and magazines with turned-down pages marking articles about the team. Rows of fat binders labeled in block letters read like a greatest hits list of atrocities. The team has searched for the disappeared in East Timor, Kosovo, Iraq, Ukraine, Kurdistan, South Africa, and many other places around the world. They investigated the disappearance of forty-three students from Ayotzinapa Rural Teachers' College in Guerrero, Mexico, at the request of the families of the missing. They exhumed the victims of notorious massacres in El Mozote, El Salvador, and Dos Erres, Guatemala. They were part of the team that recovered the remains of the Cuban-Argentine revolutionary Che Guevara in Bolivia. In Chile, they investigated the deaths of poet Pablo Neruda and politician Salvador Allende, assassinated in General Augusto Pinochet's coup. The team's expertise has been called on by the United Nations International Criminal Tribunal for the former Yugoslavia, the International Criminal Court, the International Committee of the Red Cross, and the Committee on Missing Persons in Cyprus.

I work with Emilia and Adriana, students from the University of Buenos Aires who are interning with the team. They are magnetic friends in an opposites-attract way: Adriana is tall, methodical, earnest, and dry-witted; Emilia is short, expressive, rainbow-haired, and quick to laugh. We work in what is called "the lab," but it is a homier space than the name suggests: a series of rooms with exam tables where we lay out the remains, and two sinks where we wash the bones.

Making notes on a skeletal inventory form, Adriana unzips her pencil case and pulls out a glitter pen and an eraser in the shape of a unicorn. Emilia brings intricate paper cutouts of the *Star Wars* Death Star that she made over the weekend, and we tape them to the windows of the lab. On breaks, they dash to the corner kiosko to buy candy. Their sweet-tooth proximity to girlhood contrasts with their growing forensic expertise. Adriana handles the dental pick with authority, probing for cavities and studying odontological features under a magnifying loupe. Emilia pulls apart a pupa casing she found in a skull, examining it for taphonomic clues about the timeline of decomposition and conditions of the gravesite. She mentions she has a collection of cocoons in her bedroom at home. I imagine the silky bundles among her *Star Wars* figurines, a tableau in a forensic coming-of-age story.

                                                    . . .

THE EAAF HAS long since established itself as a legendary forensic team. Since it was founded in 1984, the team has carried out hundreds of exhumations in more than sixty countries. It has offices in Buenos Aires, Mexico City, and New York, and a forensic genetics lab in the Argentine city of Córdoba, with seventy team members working in fields including forensic anthropology, archaeology, genetics, and pathology. The work they do—exhuming mass graves to investigate human rights violations—feels like such ethical common sense that it can be hard to remember that they were the first to do it. Before 1984, human rights forensics didn't exist. It all began with a group of friends Adriana and Emilia's age.

Immediately after the fall of the Argentine dictatorship in 1983, judges ordered the excavation of sections of municipal cemeteries in Buenos Aires, where the bodies of desaparecidos were believed to be buried. Heavy machinery clawed through graves, crushing bones, intermingling bodies, and destroying evidence. These calamitous exhumations, dubbed "the horror show," led human rights groups and families of the missing to seek help from experts outside the country. The newly formed truth commission, Comisión Nacional Sobre la Desaparición de Personas (CONADEP), and the Grandmothers of Plaza de Mayo (the Abuelas), a group of mothers of the disappeared searching for babies born in clandestine detention centers, contacted the American Association for the Advancement of Science (AAAS) for advice. They wanted to know how forensic science and emerging genetic research could help them find the missing and the dead, a quest that would eventually revolutionize the fields of forensics and genetics. This history offers "an alternative origin story" for these scientific advances, one led by mothers in the Global South, not scientists in the Global North, as anthropologist Lindsay A. Smith has explored in her work.

In June 1984, a delegation from AAAS arrived for a ten-day visit to Argentina. Among the scientists was Dr. Clyde Snow, a celebrated forensic pioneer known for high-profile cases like analyzing the remains of Nazi physician Josef Mengele and identifying victims of serial killers Jeffrey Dahmer and John Wayne Gacy. Snow met with human rights activists and families of the disappeared. He visited the exhumations and found them even more destructive and unscientific than expected. Plastic bags crammed with bones from several bodies gathered dust in storerooms. Hundreds of bodies had been exhumed, and none had been identified. "They were losing evidence," he said, "which is as bad as being an accomplice to the crime." Reflecting on what he'd seen, he argued that a single methodical excavation would yield more evidence of human rights abuses than a hundred reckless ones. The AAAS delegation called on the government to halt the horror show.

A young judge helping the Abuelas de Plaza de Mayo approached Dr. Snow. Judge Ramos Padilla had a lead on a clandestine burial site. Could the grave be exhumed before the delegation departed? Snow accepted the challenge and contacted local archaeologists and forensic medicine specialists for help. "I checked all around," he later said, but "none of the professional archaeologists wanted to get involved." Some declined because they were afraid. Taking part in a public attempt to find the disappeared was a risky proposition in a country known for the frequency of its military coups. Others refused because they were complicit. In Argentina, forensic experts are part of the police and judicial systems, and many had participated in the junta's crimes. Some had falsified death certificates to hide atrocities. In one dictatorship-era autopsy report, a coroner examined a body riddled with bullets and declared the cause of death "acute anemia."

With only a few days left in the AAAS delegation's visit, Snow's unofficial translator took matters into his own hands. Morris Tidball-Binz, a shaggy-haired medical student, had taken a liking to the slow-talking, fedora-wearing, chain-smoking Texan, and tried to convince his friends to help. He managed to recruit a handful of anthropology and archaeology students, including Patricia "Pato" Bernardi, Luis Fondebrider, and Mercedes "Mimi" Doretti, whose mother was a well-known journalist and part of the truth commission. They piled into two police cars for the drive to the Boulogne cemetery on the city's outskirts. They would soon form the EAAF and become the first-ever forensic team dedicated to human rights work. In a few years, Clyde Snow would call them "the most experienced team of forensic archeologists in the world." But that morning in June 1984, they were students who had grown up under a brutal military dictatorship, riding in police cars that they associated with abduction, not protection. Argentina was only six months into a fragile democracy, which was far from guaranteed to survive. They were about the same age as most of the disappeared. They understood that by searching for the missing, they would be indelibly marked. If the junta or their sympathizers returned to power, they would be the first to be sucked into secret prisons. But they wanted to do something tangible and concrete to expose the terrors they had lived through. "We didn't talk about science," says Luis Fondebrider. "It was a political act."

. . .

ONE MORNING, I arrive late to the lab. Walking to the back room, I hear water running and pop songs bubbling on the radio. Adriana and Emilia are already at work. They lean over two sinks scrubbing skulls with pink and yellow toothbrushes. In the hall, a commercial baker's cart is stacked with bones drying on cookie sheets, like pastries in a witch's bakery. *Baby, I love your way* sings the radio as Emilia slides her finger into the eye socket of a skull. I wonder what someone would think if they wandered in off the street. I suit up in a plastic apron and gloves and trade places with Emilia, who starts double-checking the racks and labels. For the next two hours, I wash bones. I wash an enormous femur, a skull splitting at the jagged sagittal suture, square facets of hamate, capitate, trapezium, and trapezoid. I wash fragments.

Every week, deliveries arrive from exhumation sites, including Pozo de Vargas. We open the large cardboard boxes to reveal dozens of sealed plastic bags labeled with information about where they were located in the excavation. The bags contain bones and bone fragments. Everything has been "cleaned in place" in the field, but there's still dirt and mud that need to be scrubbed away so the bones can be analyzed and measured. We work systematically, one bag at a time, carefully transferring labels and documenting the chain of custody. We wash about three hundred bones and bone fragments on a good day. We aren't examining or analyzing the remains at this stage. We're just cleaning. But, as you wash, you see a lot of bones. No two bodies are the same, and you learn the normal range of variation by handling bones. Distinctive marks from trauma, pathology, or postmortem damage start to jump out. Every hour or so, we discover a "feature of interest." We stop everything and bring the bone to the window for better light, inspecting it and exchanging theories. If we come across something we can't make sense of, we bring it to Cati or one of the other senior team members, who can usually explain it at a glance. Washing, while not glamorous, serves a role in forensic training. It is essential to see and touch hundreds of bones.

Few people in European and American societies touch the dead. Pathologists in the morgue, medical students in anatomy class, undertakers preparing funerals, and forensic anthropologists at exhumation sites and labs. As archaeologist Rosemary Joyce says, "We need to acknowledge that, at least in the world today, our intimate experience with the dead marks us. We are not everyday." In the forensic lab, touching bones is what we do every day. It is hands-on work. Lifting and moving the bones reveals their shapes and how they relate to one another. We use our own bodies as anatomical atlases. By holding a femur against my leg, the bones of a wrist against my wrist, or by pressing my flesh to feel my own bones, I can better visualize their position. We recognize our bodies in the skeletons and the skeletons in our bodies.

Touching bones reveals clues about age, sex, and trauma. As I struggled to articulate bones in Guatemala, José would tell me: tocar para ver—touch to see. I didn't yet understand what that meant, how the "sensual geography" of the body must be mapped through touch. Feel the pubic symphysis: Does it have the sandpaper texture of young bone, or is it smooth like older bone? Pinch the orbital ridge between your thumb and forefinger: The bone's sharpness or bluntness gives clues to sex. Press your thumb into the greater sciatic notch of the pelvis to measure its dimorphic angles. Run your fingers across the surface of a broken bone: Green bone fractures are sharp and smooth, and dry bone fractures are rough and uneven, indicating the timing of trauma.

We compare text and bones, consulting books and tables. To estimate age, the textbook *Forensic Anthropology: Current Methods and Practice* lists the six phases of sternal rib changes. Bones proceed from "a billowy, flat appearance when young, to a cupped flared shape when middle aged, to a wide shape with irregular sharp margins in advanced age." We compare these words to the fourth rib, where the bone connects to costal cartilage. Tactile knowledge is crucial for analyzing bones. Visual inspection is not enough; "it is notoriously difficult to work from photographs alone," an academic journal article on osteoarchaeology warns. Forensic textbooks mention the shapes and textures of bones but don't offer detailed instruction on haptic examination of the skeleton; touch is oddly footnoted. A forensic practitioner touches a sternal rib to understand age. Yet, in the textbook passage cited above, tactile qualities (billowy, flared, flat, sharp) are referred to as "appearance," as if they were only visual. Thus, touch is a skill that floats at the edge of forensics, crucial yet somehow disavowed.

This may be in part because of the constraints of textbooks and lectures. Touch, like taste or smell, cannot be easily printed on a page or described in a lecture. Tactile knowledge is embodied and must be experienced to be learned. But the lack of attention to touch is also a product of how the senses are culturally ranked. In European and American societies, sight dominates. Vision is closely associated with the "higher" realms of mind and intelligence. In contrast, touch is associated with the "lower" domains of the flesh, its pains and pleasures, its birthing and dying. In *The Book of Touch*, cultural historian Constance Classen writes that the "sensation of touch, like the body in general, has been positioned in opposition to the intellect." In the hierarchy of the senses, sight is lofty, and touch is base. In line with this cultural pecking order, "visual inspection" is acknowledged as a standard step in forensic analysis, but "tactile inspection," though just as crucial and just as frequently performed, is not mentioned.

Smooth, rough, pitted, granular, gritty, rugged, ridged, undulating, grooved, sharp, creased, curved—the shapes and textures of bone carry messages for those who can read them. The art of forensic touch is honed through years of practice.

. . .

WHEN CLYDE SNOW and the students arrived at the Boulogne cemetery in San Isidro, they were greeted by Judge Ramos Padilla and his entourage. Dozens of police arrived, followed by a police physician wearing a camel hair coat. Soon more than forty officials had gathered by the grave—who among them had been complicit in disappearances? Snow instructed Morris, the medical student, and the others to stake out a perimeter around the grave. Then, flashing his coroners association badge, Snow announced that only the judge and the forensic team would be allowed to access the grave. The police protested, but Judge Padilla agreed. Snow later told a journalist, "I always carry it around, because whenever you get into a confrontation with police, the guy with the biggest badge wins." It was a trick he'd use again in Guatemala when he trained the forensic team there a few years later.

They were searching for the remains of Rosa Rufina Betti de Casagrande, who had disappeared in November 1976. Judge Padilla had received credible information that Rosa had been buried in an unmarked grave, known in Argentina as N.N. (ningún nombre, or no name). Clyde Snow was showing the students how to determine the depth of the grave by digging a test probe when

Rosa's mother and father arrived. Snow was taken aback; in the United States, families would never be allowed at a crime scene. In Argentina, things were different. Families of the missing had spearheaded the search for the disappeared. Protests held by mothers of the disappeared had brought the junta's human rights abuses to international attention. It was the Abuelas de Plaza de Mayo who had invited the AAAS delegation and who were working with Judge Padilla to investigate cases. The presence of Rosa's family at the grave may have shocked Snow, but it didn't surprise the students. It made sense to them. "It was totally driven by the families," Luis Fondebrider tells me. From the beginning, exhumations were one piece of a much bigger project of restoring democracy and creating new forms of transparency and accountability after tyranny. When the students searched for Rosa, they were taking part in a collective effort by families, human rights activists, lawyers, artists—an entire society—to grapple with the atrocities of the dictatorship. Clyde Snow knew the science, but the students understood the political importance of what they were doing.

. . .

IN THE EAAF lab, Adriana clamps a femur to a stool and plugs in the electric saw. "Watch your hair," says Emilia, gesturing at Adriana's long braid, which dangles precariously close to the blade. Adriana tosses her hair behind her back. She fires up the saw and the lights dim. The whole setup makes me nervous. The stool is rickety, and Adriana awkwardly steadies it with her foot. The bone doesn't fit securely in the clamp because it isn't square; it has a slight helix twist. She seems nervous and hesitant. She brings the blade down onto the bone. It slips off.

Samples can most reliably be taken from the femur, tibia, or tooth, or, if those are missing, the pelvis. The goal is to remove a small rectangle of bone sufficient to extract DNA. Family members must be warned about the sample. Otherwise, they may see the missing piece and think it is evidence of terrible torture. Cati tells me that she once forgot to warn a mother who was deeply troubled by the wound in the bone. "You only forget once," she says. The tricky part is to remove only a piece of the bone and not accidentally cut it in half. That would be a disaster. How would you explain that to a family?

Maybe the blade is dull, or the angle is awkward, or Adriana is simply inexperienced, but the initial cut eludes her. The blade keeps slipping, and Emilia and I are getting tense. "With more force!" says Emilia. I can tell she wants to intervene. She is more experienced at DNA samples, but to interrupt Adriana would be to call her competence into question.

At last, the blade bites into the bone. The motor slows, and dust rises. It smells like burning hair. Emilia pulls the bandanna she is wearing around her neck over her nose. The smell is a reminder that the bone is not a stick; this is not a carpentry project. The odor is biological and violent.

. . .

OCCASIONALLY, THE BONES smell faintly of decay. The distinctive odor is from compounds called cadaverine and putrescine, also found in urine and semen. When you smell decomposition, it is because particles with a precise molecular weight and a simple zigzag structure have entered your body through your nose, that is, through a hole in your skull. The senses are a function of our biological porosity.

We handle the bones carefully because they are fragile, but we are fragile, too. Human remains are potential vectors of contagion. Clean and dry bones pose little risk, but "wet bodies" and gravesites are another matter. Alvaro, of the Guatemalan team, was hospitalized with an infection of his inner ear that threatened his hearing, acquired from contact with decomposing bodies. After that, he always wore gloves when handling bones, but this is unusual. Seeing Alvaro rebuffed when he tried to share gloves with other team members, I asked him about it. He said, "They don't think it can happen to them, even though lots of them have problems from handling the bodies."

"Like what?" I asked.

"Problems with their skin, things like that." As one textbook says, forensic anthropology often has an "ethos of disregard, indeed disdain for health and safety procedures." Alvaro said that Clyde Snow had warned him that spores can survive fifty years in graves and make you sick. Infection travels with touch and smell, unlike with other senses.

In the lab, we work with clean bones, using our bare hands to better feel their textures and read their surfaces. Handling bones can leave traces of DNA from sweat, oil, and tiny flakes of skin, and samples must be carefully prepared before genetic testing to avoid contamination. The living must be protected from the dead, but the bones must be protected from us, too.

．　．　．

AFTER TEN MINUTES of careful sawing, Adriana extracts a rectangle of bone about five inches long and two inches wide. She holds it above her head in a teasing victory stance, but she is clearly a little shaken. "You did good," says Emilia. She pulls a pack of cigarettes from her bag and offers one to Adriana. They lean out the window to smoke, watching the traffic.

Another day, I extract a sample. It is not technically complex, and I saw out the piece without a problem, but I don't like doing it. After all the time and care to excavate bones, wash the smallest fragments, and puzzle them together, it feels wrong to cut one apart.

Later, in the genetics lab, the bone samples will be reduced to fragments for DNA extraction. There are special grinders for this, but it can also be done by placing the bone on an anvil and beating it with a hammer. "It feels bad to do it," Noelia, a lab technician, told me. "But it must be done." With this, Noelia folded the hood of her hazmat suit over her head, tucked away her long hair, adjusted her mask and safety glasses, and brought down the hammer.

The bones of a skeleton have recognizable humanity. But once the sample is cut away, it becomes a thing: a rigid rectangle hardly distinguishable from a scrap of wood or plastic. Pulverized, it loses all connection to a person. Yet, from this dust, identity will be restored. The sample will reveal genetic codes and lead to family members. Through scientific identification, bones that are now marked with a series of numbers will regain names. And with a name, a body can be given a proper burial. From dust to dust.

. . .

AT THE BOULOGNE cemetery in San Isidro, Clyde Snow directed the search for Rosa's body. After about an hour of digging, the dirt changed color. Working gently and slowly, trying to look more confident than they felt, the fledgling team scraped away the soil. Snow was proud of this "very gallant little group of Argentine anthropology and medical students." He instructed them as they improvised with their rudimentary tools. They used a window screen that Luis had "borrowed" from his mother's house as a sieve to sift through the dirt for fragments of bones, teeth, and bullets, and dug with a teaspoon they had pressed into service as a trowel.

Morris was standing in the grave scraping dirt when he uncovered bone. Snow knew this was a critical moment. How would the young team react to the body? Morris worked intently using the teaspoon to expose part of a gracile skull. An earthworm was stuck to the bone. Pato, one of the anthropology students, turned white, scrambled out of the grave, and ran away. Snow found her kneeling behind a parked car, crying. His motto was "work in the day and cry at night," but he knew not everyone was cut out for the forensic trade. He worried Pato's reaction was a bad sign. He thought, "Once this kind of thing gets started, it'll spread, and they'll decide this is not the kind of thing they want to do." Fifteen minutes later, Pato came back to the excavation. Standing at the edge of the grave, she said, "Morris, give me the spoon."

"What do you want the spoon for?" he asked.

"I'm going to make coffee."

Relating this story to a journalist, Snow said, "That's when I figured, well, maybe we've got a team."

. . .

IN THE AFTERNOONS, as we work in the lab, we drink yerba mate. The bitter tea, prepared in a gourd and sipped through a metal straw, is a social drink, always shared. As we analyze bones, we pass the gourd from person to person. The configuration of the tables and the arrangement of the bones means that the yerba mate often rests by the hands of the skeleton as if they, too, are taking part in the ritual. This is sometimes a source of jokes.

"Che, stop hogging the yerba mate!" Adriana says when Emilia hasn't passed the cup.

"Don't blame me; it's this guy's fault!" says Emilia, gesturing to the skeleton in front of her. "He takes forever to drink it." The humor is gentle and affectionate. I wanted to write "ribbing between friends," an unintentional pun when the friends are ribs. With teaspoons and yerba mate gourds, through jokes and tears, the bones shift between people and evidence.

· · ·

IN COURTROOM TRIALS, forensic scientists testify, explaining to lawyers and judges how bones offer evidence of human rights abuses. Yet exhumation exists precisely because bones are missing people, searched for and grieved by families and communities. These two aspects, evidence and personhood, are inseparable and can come into tension. A mass grave can attest to atrocity without each body being identified. Such an exhumation would be useful in a human rights trial but of little help for a family searching for a loved one. A body can be returned to a family, but if there is no trial, it will be of little use for proving crimes against humanity. If a forensic anthropologist cries and runs away while exhuming a skull, she will do her job poorly. But if she cares so little that she shovels the bones like sticks, she will also do her job poorly.

If you can't understand the bones as people who are missed and loved, with a mother and father standing by the edge of the grave waiting, you can't do this work. If you can't understand the bones as evidence to be analyzed and examined, you can't do this work. You must touch bones and be touched by them. You must be able to drink your tea with the dead.

· · ·

CLYDE SNOW GUIDED the team through the exhumation. When the cranium was unearthed, they could see a bullet hole above the eye. As more of the remains were revealed, Snow knew it was the skeleton of a young woman, which meant it might be Rosa.

After seven hours, as the sun set, they photographed the fully exposed skeleton and gently removed the bones from the soggy dirt. In the winter darkness, they drove to the San Isidro morgue.

They cleaned the bones in an exam room, arranging them on an autopsy table while Rosa's mother and father waited in the hall.

They had no dental records or radiographs to work with, and genetic testing didn't exist yet. Analyzing and measuring the bones, Snow worked to determine sex, age, stature, and trauma. Looking on, the police physician wearing a camel hair coat insisted that the injuries were consistent with an armed encounter, echoing the junta's stories of terrorists killed in gun battles with the military. Snow replied that the bones would tell.

Just before 2:00 A.M., Snow left the exam room to talk to Rosa's family. With Morris translating, he said that the probable cause of death was a single close-range gunshot wound, consistent with an execution, not a shoot-out. But the murdered young woman was not their daughter. The forensic findings were inconsistent with her height and age. Rosa's mother began to cry. The team did, too. It was a strange conclusion to a long day. There was little hope that Rosa was alive, and another mother's daughter lay on the autopsy table. Yet the excavation demonstrated that forensic science could be applied to finding Argentina's disappeared. It proved that the nascent team could do the work.

⋅ ⋅ ⋅

OVER THE NEXT year, the team exhumed hundreds of N.N. graves. In April 1985, a landmark human rights trial began. General Videla and eight other junta leaders faced 711 charges ranging from forgery to kidnapping, torture, and murder. Clyde Snow presented forensic evidence at "Argentina's Nuremberg," as the press referred to the proceedings.

In his testimony, Snow focused on the case of a young woman named Liliana Carmen Pereyra, whose remains the team had recently exhumed. The military presented its standard story, claiming that she was a guerrilla fighter, killed in a shoot-out. Telling the judges that "the skeleton is its own best witness," Snow projected an image of Liliana's skull on a large screen in the courtroom. Her cranium had been shattered into twenty pieces, which, glued back into place, clearly revealed a gunshot wound. The case had "all the markings of an execution," said Snow, describing the evidence as consistent with a close-range gunshot. "That's tough to do in an armed encounter unless only one side is armed," he told the court in his Texas drawl.

The forensic evidence presented in Liliana's case was crucial to the verdict. The judges found the junta guilty of human rights violations and sentenced General Jorge Videla to life in prison. The convictions cleared the way for a "justice cascade" of similar trials in Latin America.

But Liliana's case was important for other reasons, too. Before the trial, soon after the team had identified Liliana from dental records, her mother, Coqui, arrived unannounced at their make-shift lab with her two teenage children in tow. They wanted to see Liliana's body. The team found an empty room and arranged Liliana's bones on a table, debating the best way to present them. They settled on separating them into tidy piles—all the bones of the arms, the legs, the ribs, and so on. Inviting Coqui and the children to see the remains, Snow explained the process of forensic identification. Eric Stover, an original member of the AAAS delegation, translated into Spanish. In Stover's words, "It was fairly clinical until the daughter reached over and grabbed her mother and gave her a big hug. The whole room dissolved into tears." Snow cried more than anyone. So much for "work in the day and cry at night."

Coqui's desire to visit Liliana's body inspired the new team to adopt the practice of inviting families to see the recovered remains if they so wished. Liliana's case made it evident that bones could be witnesses in trials and offer solace to the grieving. Justice and care became the double helix of EAAF's forensic practices.

You could say that the Argentine forensic team is in its third generation now. Clyde Snow trained the students who formally became the EAAF in May 1987. Its founding members were Morris Tidball-Binz, Patricia Bernardi, Mercedes Doretti, Luis Fondebrider, Alejandro Incháurregui, and Darío Olmo. Clyde Snow was appointed an honorary member. The original team now teaches students like Adriana and Emilia. Mimi's mother was part of the CONADEP truth commission, and Emilia's father was one of the early members of the EAAF. Morris, Pato, Mimi, Luis, and the others who first formed the team were the same age as the disappeared, and now children of desaparecidos work on the team.

In these generations of working intimately with the dead, the team has learned forensic touch: the tactile clues bones offer and how to bring a human touch to the work, excavating with families at the graveside and inviting them into the lab. Reflecting on the earliest exhumations of the EAAF, Luis Fondebrider says, "We had a relationship with the relatives of the disappeared from the beginning. We were the same age as their children when they disappeared and they had a special affection for us." He adds, "And then there was the fact that we touched their dead. Touching the dead creates a special relationship with people."

When families come to the lab to see the remains of their loved ones, they sometimes touch and kiss the bones. Berta Schubaroff, a mother of a desaparecido and a member of the Abuelas de Plaza de Mayo, described receiving the remains of her son, Marcelo Gelman: "I began to kiss him, kiss all of his bones, touch him, and caress him." The bones are the beloved.

Once I watched Cati measure a cranial fracture. When she finished, she ran her palm along the frontal bone, touching the skull just like you'd stroke a sick kid's forehead. It was an action with no scientific purpose, an unmistakable gesture of comfort. She did it without thinking. I could have easily missed her fleeting touch, distracted by studying the fracture pattern. Or I could have seen it but not registered its significance because I already "knew" what she was doing: analyzing a bullet trajectory, not comforting someone. My feeling of surprise could have dispersed without a trace. But I caught it and afterward noticed many subtle and ephemeral touches of care: adjusting the angle of bones to a more "comfortable" position, patting a skull and saying "pobrecito."

"The first thing I do with the bones is touch them," Pato explained, many years after the first muddy exhumation in Boulogne cemetery. Forensic teams touch bones to exhume remains, wash the mud from fragments, glue a fractured skull, saw out a DNA sample, feel the texture of fractures, and sometimes to comfort the dead.

CHAPTER 9

Mothers

ANA MARÍA CAREAGA BURSTS THROUGH the door of the faculty lounge, wearing a red leather jacket and a rainbow scarf. She immediately makes a joke about being late with a big laugh. It is a strange feeling to know intimate details about someone's life before you've met them—about the scars on their body documented by human rights groups and their grief described by journalists. But almost instantly, this vanishes into another kind of intimacy—the affinity of meeting someone magnetic and wanting to know them.

Ana María teaches at the University of Buenos Aires. She is a psychoanalyst, a former director of Instituto Espacio para la Memoria, and an internationally known human rights activist. She is one of the few survivors of the clandestine detention centers, and her testimony has been crucial in documenting the atrocities of the dictatorship. Her story is well known. She regularly gives public lectures and speaks with the media. Another activist gave me her number. I was nervous about calling. I spent hours carefully preparing my interview questions. I arrived early at the psychology department, with its worn façade, creaking pipes suspended from the ceilings, and cheerful corridors papered with posters and flyers. Passing the time wandering the halls, I came across a list of disappeared faculty and students affixed to a wall.

As Ana María and I walk through the neighborhood, we fall into deep conversation about the possibilities of memory, justice, and repair, my carefully prepared questions forgotten. She tells me about a course she is teaching on the intersection of human rights and psychoanalysis. She emphasizes the importance of recognizing the individual amid universalizing ideas. We talk about understanding the "human" in human rights. "Otherwise," she says, "it all becomes an abstraction."

On June 13, 1977, Ana María was standing at the busy intersection of Juan B. Justo and Corrientes streets in Buenos Aires. A car pulled to the curb, and before she had time to react, two men in civilian clothes grabbed her and shoved her inside. They pushed her down onto the backseat and blindfolded her. They brought her to a building; through a small gap at the bottom of the blindfold, she could see car tires and that the men around her wore black boots with blue uniform pants tucked into them. She could smell grease and engine oil. She was forced down a ladder into a basement. She was at "Club Atlético," a notorious secret prison in the bowels of a federal police building.

. . .

ANA MARÍA'S MOTHER, Esther Ballestrino de Careaga, began a desperate search for her daughter. Their family had already been touched by disappearance. Manuel Carlos Cuevas, the husband of Ana María's sister Mabel, had been taken. The couple was expecting a child. Esther visited prisons, police stations, hospitals, and churches, looking for information and help. Every door was closed in her face. During this quest, she met other mothers searching for their own missing children. When Ana María was taken, Esther sought out these women.

The mothers met every week. It started with fourteen women. "Where should we meet?" Somewhere public, where people would notice them. "What time?" "Well, after cooking for the family, after cleaning the kitchen, before they close the banks." On Saturday, April 30, 1977, less than two months before Ana

María's abduction, the mothers arrived at the Plaza de Mayo, a public square in front of Casa Rosada, Argentina's pink stone presidential palace. But the plaza was nearly empty because few people came downtown on the weekends. The next time, they met on a Friday, but one of the mothers said Fridays were unlucky, that it was the day of witches. So they settled on Thursdays at 3:30 in the afternoon.

Every week they gathered to demand information about their missing children. "We wore flat shoes so we could make a run for it if they came for us." Most of the mothers had no political experience. They were housewives, factory workers, cleaners, and teachers. Esther was different. She and her husband, Raymundo Dejesús, were politically experienced activists. They fled Paraguay's military dictatorship in the late 1940s and settled in Buenos Aires. Just before Ana María's abduction, Raymundo had been writing a human rights report that was taken from his desk during a raid on the family's home. Esther was an outspoken feminist who had been a leader in the fight for women's rights in Paraguay. She had a doctorate in biochemistry and pharmacology, and ran a lab.

The Madres de Plaza de Mayo learned as they went. At first, they sat on benches scattered around the square. They alerted one another to their sisterhood by holding twigs and pinning tree leaves to their collars. They hid slips of paper in balls of wool and knit scarves on park benches, passing notes. They made plans. They printed decals and leaflets, discreetly leaving them on buses and subways. They wrote messages on peso notes, hoping they would be read as people paid for newspapers that never mentioned the disappearances or magazines with cover photos of the dictator Videla and his wife playing with their young children.

When the mothers bought newspapers, it was to roll them up and swat the police dogs that were sometimes unleashed on them in the plaza. The junta had outlawed meetings of more than three people, and as the group got larger and more conspicuous, the police became more aggressive. They shooed the Madres off the benches. *Why?* they asked; it was a public place, and there were many people there. The police conceded this was true, but everyone else was walking. And so, they walked, counterclockwise around the square, "as if rebelling against every minute without their children," as if to undo time.

When Ana María was abducted, Esther and the Madres went to the only newspaper that regularly reported on disappearances, the *Buenos Aires Herald*, a small English-language daily. The first week after the coup, the junta issued a decree forbidding the press from promoting news or opinions "lessening the prestige of the activities of the Armed Forces." A later statement declared, "As from today it is forbidden to comment or make references to suspects connected with subversive incidents, the appearance of bodies and the deaths of subversive elements." The *Buenos Aires Herald* printed the text of this prohibition on its front page in protest, but only one other newspaper mentioned it. Those defying censorship would be "subject to detention for a period of up to ten years." The actual punishment being more lethal, of course. Journalists were particular targets for disappearance. Jacobo Timerman, the editor of the influential paper *La Opinión*, characterized it as a "genocide of journalists." Timerman was kidnapped in April 1977 and held in a secret detention center. Because he was a high-profile figure, international pressure eventually led to his release. From exile, he wrote the bestselling book *Prisoner Without a Name, Cell Without a Number*, a detailed account of his torture and imprisonment, revealing the Nazi sympathies of his captors. Published in 1981, it gave one of the most important early accounts of the atrocities being committed by the junta.

Even as the military kidnapped and killed journalists, Robert

Cox, the editor of the *Buenos Aires Herald*, refused to be silenced. Cox had grown up in England during the Second World War, and while he initially supported the junta, he soon began to see disturbing parallels between Argentina and Nazi Germany. "It was an honour to scream when everybody else held silence," he said. But speaking out put Cox, his family, and the journalists he worked with in danger.

Esther met with Cox to discuss the delicate question of whether to publish a story about Ana María's abduction. On rare occasions, people held in clandestine detention centers were allowed to call or visit their families, proof that some people survived long after they were abducted. Some prisoners were even released, adding to the sense of uncertainty. The terror and ambiguity of El Proceso kept families quiet—who would dare agitate, knowing that your son or daughter might still be alive and anything you said could get them killed? Esther and Cox debated: If Ana María were still alive, would media attention put her at greater risk? Would she be killed to silence Esther and the Madres? Or would attention help get her released? They decided that publicizing Ana María's case was the best option, and the *Herald* reported her disappearance.

. . .

AT CLUB ATLÉTICO, Ana María's abductors ordered her to take off her clothes. They threw her to the ground, stepped on her wrists to hold her down, and poured buckets of water over her. She struggled to breathe under the deluge. They demanded information about her family. Then they took her to the quirofano, the "operating room," as they called it, where they tortured people. The pain from the picana, the electric cattle prod, was overwhelming, and she passed out.

What they did in the quirofano wasn't the only form of torture. They offered her a cup of tea at the end of the first torture session. She was cold and thirsty, but as she reached for the yerba mate, they told her that drinking liquid after the electric shocks might stop her heart. She was forbidden to say her name; they gave her a code. "I was K04," she tells me. "They took away my name." Ana María found, "There are all kinds of people in the camp, the demagogues, the torturers." There is the sadist "who enjoys the suffering, screams, and pain of the tortured." But there are also "the impeccably dressed gentlemen who come to see how things are. All they do is observe, and ask 'How old are you?' 'Sixteen, sir.' 'Did they torture you?' 'Yes, sir.' And he looks at the marks on your body and goes away."

In the torture sessions that followed, the men sought out the most sensitive areas of her body: eyes, ears, vagina. They applied electric shocks and poured kerosene on tender skin. They suspended her by her arms from ropes until her skin peeled away. When they noticed she was trying to control the pain by holding her breath, they accused her of doing "yoga" and put a sheet of plastic over her nose and mouth so that she could not breathe. This was called the "dry submarine" and proved fatal for some prisoners. Although the pain was so great that she often lost consciousness, and although she heard the cries of other prisoners being tortured, she didn't scream. "I don't know why I didn't, but it infuriated them." They tortured her more. On the third day, she gave the torturers her family's address. She calculated that her parents would have already gone into hiding. When they discovered the house empty, they were irate. They tortured her more.

. . .

AFTER ANA MARÍA'S abduction, Esther called a former employee, a young chemistry technician named Jorge Bergoglio, who had worked in her lab. Despite their many differences—they were twenty years apart in age; she performed immaculate tests

in the lab, he was a bit sloppy; he was a priest, she was a Marxist—
they had become close friends. On the phone, Esther asked him
to come quickly; her mother-in-law was dying and needed last
rites. He hurried to Esther's house, puzzled because he knew
that Esther wasn't religious. When Bergoglio arrived, he learned
the true nature of the summons. Would he hide their books?
Their leftist library was a dangerous liability. Bergoglio agreed.

Many of the Madres were devoutly religious, and the church
was the first place they went for help finding their children. They
were turned away. On the rare occasions when the mothers were
received, priests did little more than promise to pray the Lord's
Prayer for the disappeared. "That was the total interview—that
they would pray for our children," related one mother. "The
Catholic Church turned its back on us." In one case, the young
son of a disappeared father wrote "a very pretty letter, a child's
letter" to a bishop, who wrote back to say it was a "decision of
God his father had disappeared and he should accept it." Madres
managed to get messages to Pope John Paul II on at least two
occasions. But when the pope visited Argentina in 1982, he refused to meet with any human rights organizations, citing a lack
of time. Lawyer and human rights activist Emilio Mignone, a
committed Catholic whose daughter Mónica was disappeared
along with several co-workers and priests while volunteering in
Bajo Flores villa, came to see the church establishment as a "web
of mediocrity, cowardice, and complicity."

In October 1977, a group of Madres met at the annual Luján
pilgrimage, which attracted thousands of believers. It was one of
the few public gatherings allowed during the dictatorship and
offered a chance to safely meet. To find one another in the crowd,
they decided to wear headscarves. *Let's use cloth baby diapers,*
suggested one mother, and so they adopted their iconic white
scarves.

Azucena Villaflor emerged as a natural leader of the Madres.

She was courageous, energetic, and well liked. She had only an elementary school education and had started working as a telephone operator at sixteen. Azucena married a trade-union worker, Pedro De Vicenti, and they had four children. Her son Néstor was abducted in November 1976.

A Madre named Chicha Mariani tells a story about meeting Azucena. Desperate to draw international attention to the plight of their children, the Madres had prepared a letter to give to U.S. Secretary of State Cyrus Vance when he visited Argentina in the spring of 1977. Chicha was selected to present the document. The Madres saw their chance as Vance paid an official visit to a public monument. But Chicha got so nervous that she froze, and he walked right by her, vanishing into a crowd of soldiers. Azucena grabbed the paper, pushed her way through the soldiers, and handed it to Vance. "That day, Azucena showed me that we were capable of doing things that we could never have imagined," said Chicha.

The mothers quickly became brave and bold. A Madre named Dora de Bazze made a huge banner out of bedsheets and broomsticks, painted with the words "Where are the detained-disappeared?" and signed "the Madres." She wrapped it to look like an ordinary package and made her way to Plaza de Mayo by subway. The Madres had never used banners because it was very dangerous, but when Dora told the other mothers, they said, "Let's open it!" They unfurled it. The military immediately came over and started kicking the mothers. Breaking one of the broomsticks, a soldier taunted, "Now what are you going to do with it?" Dora wielded the broken broom and responded, "Stick it up your ass!" The thirty or forty mothers gathered began to shout, "Where are our children?" facing a line of soldiers with truncheons and machine guns.

The police often harassed and detained the Madres. When one Madre was asked for her papers, every Madre at the square would offer their documents, foisting ID cards at the police until the scene attracted attention from passersby. When one Madre was detained, all the Madres showed up at the police station insisting on being arrested, too. Once, so many women demanded to be arrested that the police had to commandeer a city bus to take them to the station. At the station, the mothers would shout, "Aren't you ashamed? Take off your uniforms, you vermin!" Then they would loudly pray Hail Marys. The police called them "the crazy women of Plaza de Mayo." This is what the press called them, too. And the junta. And many of their neighbors and friends.

Women who had been afraid to hand a sheet of paper to a politician confronted soldiers armed with machine guns. Women who had once had little knowledge of politics became sophisticated strategists. They had become the political activists the military accused their children of being. "Our children gave birth to us," the Madres say.

. . .

IN HER SECOND month of captivity at Club Atlético, Ana María felt her baby move for the first time. She was three months pregnant at the time of her abduction, but she hid it from her captors until she started to show. Later, European human rights lawyers investigating Ana María's case asked why she didn't reveal the pregnancy right away, naïvely believing this would have granted her better treatment. But Ana María knew better. Pregnancy was no shield against abuse, and often "the regime's depravity reached its outer limit with pregnant detainees," as Marguerite Feitlowitz observed. Once Ana María's pregnancy was known, they beat her for having hid it. They tortured her in new ways, kicking her in the stomach and threatening to tear the baby out of her belly.

Ana María began to think that she was alive in a nightmare.

That this was not life at all, but some other dimension. Once when she was alone with a doctor in the infirmary, he took off her blindfold and told her to look at the sunlight. Through small gaps, "I could hear people walking by, cars and buses passing, life going on as usual." It seemed impossible that another life was so close. "We were in the world but not part of it, alive in the realm of death." After soccer games, from her cell, she could hear fans celebrating in the street and car horns blowing. Meanwhile, the guards played cards and listened to a cassette tape of Hitler's speeches. When the torturers took breaks from the "operating room," they played Ping-Pong.

Ana María was terrified that she had lost her pregnancy because of the torture. "I was lying down in the cell . . . and suddenly she started to move: It was the only time I cried in the concentration camp," she tells me. Alone in her cell, Ana María spoke to her baby, making up poems for her, caressing her belly. "It was a triumph in that place of death, that there was life, and that there was a place where they had not been able to get to."

Her baby "had fought death," and this offered Ana María a kind of hope. "I had to resist for her and with her," she tells me. A month later, the guards entered her cell, blindfolded her, and shoved her into a car. After a drive through city traffic, the door opened, and they pushed her out. The car drove off. She looked around and realized she was a block away from her house.

. . .

ANA MARÍA TELLS me, "My reunion with my mother was a powerful thing, one of the most important things of my life." She describes her release from Club Atlético as we sit at a sidewalk table at the café we've found after a long walk through the neighborhood. She had been detained for nearly four months. She was seven months pregnant by the time she was freed. Esther quickly made arrangements to take her daughters to Brazil. They were granted protection by the United Nations high commissioner and soon accepted as political refugees by Sweden.

Ana María, Mabel, and Mabel's son Carlos traveled to Stockholm, where they were eventually joined by their older sister. But their mother did not come with them. Esther immediately returned to Buenos Aires. When she arrived at the weekly march at the Plaza de Mayo, the other mothers were shocked to see her. Her daughter had been found; why had she come back? Esther replied that she would stay and fight for all the missing. "I'll continue until they all appear, because all the disappeared are my children," she said. Ana María says, "You see, it had already gone from being an individual search to becoming a collective demand." It was bigger than any of them; it was a social movement. Ana María unwraps her rainbow scarf and waves down the kid working behind the counter. She tells me that the military wanted to put a stop to the Madres. From the beginning, it was clear that the "crazy women of Plaza de Mayo" were a powerful adversary. The Thursday protests that had started with fourteen women now filled the square. The junta wanted to "dismantle the movement, of course," says Ana María. Military leaders devised a scheme: They would infiltrate the Madres.

• • •

THE *BUENOS AIRES HERALD* carried news about disappearances, but the Madres needed more people to know. They had to get their story into one of the big Spanish-language papers read by porteños every morning. Since the newspapers refused to cover the abductions, the Madres decided they would buy space to publicize their search for their missing children. In the summer of 1977, Esther, Azucena, and the other founding mothers began to quietly raise money to run a full-page notice on December 10, International Human Rights Day, listing the names of the disappeared. *La Nación*, a major paper, agreed to publish it.

On December 8, the Madres gathered at Iglesia Santa Cruz, one of the few places that had opened its doors to them and offered them a regular place to meet. It was Día de la Virgen, a holy day in the Catholic year and a holiday in Argentina. The church was crowded. The Madres met in the garden to pool the money they had collected. Just after 8:00 P.M., a military "task force" burst onto the church grounds. They grabbed the Madres, shouting that it was a drug raid, pulling the women by their clothes and hair into cars double-parked on the street. María Eugenia Ponce de Bianco, Esther Ballestrino de Careaga, Angela Auad, Patricia Cristina Oviedo, Raquel Bulit, Eduardo Gabriel Horane, and Sister Alice Domon, a French nun working with the Madres, were taken. The same day, Remo Carlos Berardo, José Julio Fondovila, and Horacio Aníbal Elbert were abducted from other places. Two days later, Azucena Villaflor was seized while shopping near her house. Sister Léonie Duquet, a friend of Sister Alice's, was also kidnapped. The Madres and their allies who were disappeared between December 8 and 10 came to be known as "the twelve of Santa Cruz."

. . .

IN THE CAFÉ, Ana María says that we'll meet at Iglesia Santa Cruz next time. She says that I have to see the church to really understand what happened. It is closed for renovation, but she can get us in anyway. She strips the paper wrapper off the straw and tells me, "It was Alfredo Astiz who infiltrated the Madres, under the name 'Gustavo Niño,' pretending to be the brother of a desaparecido."

. . .

NAVY INTELLIGENCE OFFICER Alfredo Astiz was known as "the Blond Angel of Death." Many of the mothers were very fond of the sweet-faced boy they knew as Gustavo, who was the same age as their missing sons. They were charmed by the kid who always wore the same blue sweater, who was so desperate to find his missing brother, and whose mother was too sick to come to the marches at Plaza de Mayo. The first Thursday afternoon he went to the square, he hung back, seemingly hesitant and afraid, before speaking to the Madres. He spent months getting close to the mothers, earning their trust. "He looks like an angel!" Sister Alice told friends. He hung on Azucena and called her frequently, which made him seem like a lost boy.

Once, at the Plaza de Mayo, the police rushed the Madres, and Gustavo threw himself into the fray with his fists raised. The mothers surrounded him in a circle to protect him, afraid he would be detained. They did not know it was a staged attack, designed to win their trust. The mothers told him it was too dangerous for a young man to be an activist, but he insisted. He never missed a march. After meetings, he always offered to drive people home. How kind, what good manners. *Where do you live?* he'd ask, opening the passenger door of his car.

"Gustavo" even raised money for the ad. He arrived at the Iglesia Santa Cruz just before eight o'clock to drop off his contribution. Before leaving, he kissed the Madres goodbye on the cheek, marking those mothers who were to be taken with a Judas kiss, as his confederates lingered nearby, watching for this sign.

The abductors took the kidnapped women to the clandestine detention center ESMA. Another prisoner crossed paths with Sister Alice there. Torture had left her arms purple with bruises, and she could barely walk. Sister Alice asked for any news of the kidnapped Madres and asked after Gustavo, the "young blond boy," worried that he had been captured, too.

The *Buenos Aires Herald* announced the abductions from Iglesia Santa Cruz in a headline on December 10, 1977, the first newspaper in Argentina to report the story. The fate of the kid-napped French nuns soon attracted international media cover-age. For the first time, the world seemed to be paying attention to the crimes taking place in Argentina. With the eyes of the world on them, military officials claimed the women had been captured by guerrillas. They released a photo of the nuns posing under a Montoneros banner. The crude forgery was taken in the basement of the secret prison and circulated widely in the press.

After the abductions, Gustavo Niño returned to Plaza de Mayo for the regular Thursday march. He approached a mother wait-ing at a café, but she told him to run away lest he be abducted like the others. Another Madre saw him gesturing to her from a street corner as if he wanted to tell her something.

Astiz continued his infiltrations, next in Europe, where he presented himself as "Eduardo Escudero" to exiled activists liv-ing in Paris. He never missed an art exhibit; he loved Calder and Van Gogh. How cultured, what an interesting young man. After meetings, he invited people to his apartment. When his cover was blown by someone who recognized him as Gustavo Niño, he escaped to Germany and eventually returned to Buenos Aires. It wasn't until the end of the dictatorship that his crimes came to light. He was deployed in the Malvinas (Falkland Islands) War, and a journalist snapped a picture of him surrendering to the British on April 26, 1982. International news agencies circulated stories about the photogenic Argentine Navy officer's capture. Recognizing the sailor as the Blond Angel of Death, France re-quested his extradition from Britain to stand trial for his role in the disappearances of French nuns Alice Domon and Léonie Du-quet. Sweden followed suit for his role in the disappearance of an Argentine-Swedish teenager named Dagmar Hagelin, whom Astiz had shot in the head when she tried to run away during a kidnap-ping. Prisoners at ESMA testified to seeing Dagmar there, her head wrapped in bandages and unable to talk. Then she disappeared. Margaret Thatcher refused the requests and sent Astiz back to Argentina, where he was frequently spotted dancing in Buenos Aires nightclubs, skiing in Bariloche, and playing polo.

Astiz's impunity lasted until 2011, when Argentine courts sentenced him to life in prison for crimes against humanity. He claimed he was just following orders. He said, "I might have made some small mistakes but for the big things I don't repent anything." Admiral Horacio Mayorga testified, "People are frightened and amazed by the Astiz affair. Do you know how many men like Astiz there were in the Navy? Three hundred Astizes." A former classmate of Astiz's observed, "He's not on the margin of the Navy. He *is* the Navy." When Astiz appeared in court for the hearings on his human rights abuses, he carried a book. It was a paperback copy of Kafka's *The Trial—El Proceso*.

The infiltration of the Madres was meant to deal the group a death blow. By destroying their leadership and killing "the best of the mothers," the military thought they would terrify and silence the others. At first, it seemed like it had worked. Only a handful of women dared to show up at Plaza de Mayo in the weeks after the abductions. But they went on. They ran the notice in *La Nación*. "For a Christmas in Peace. We only ask for the truth," it said. ("Gustavo Niño" was among the signatures published.) On Thursdays, the circle of women wearing white headscarves and marching around the plaza grew larger and larger. The disappearances of the Madres did not break them; it only strengthened their determination. "They thought there was only one Azucena, but there wasn't just one. There were hundreds of us."

• • •

ANA MARÍA AND I have been talking for nearly two hours. She answers a call from her daughter, and when she hangs up, she says, "It sounds strange now, but back then, there weren't cell-phones or anything like that." She was granted two telephone calls when she arrived in Sweden as a refugee. She used the first to tell her mother they had reached Stockholm safely and saved the second for the baby's birth. On December 11, 1977, she phoned her mother to tell her that she'd delivered a baby girl. When the call connected to Buenos Aires, she learned that Esther had been kidnapped three days earlier.

"In those three days, the two most important things in my life happened. My daughter was born, and my mother—" she breaks off. "I didn't have the chance to tell her that my daughter was born healthy and well."

CHAPTER 10

Seven Griefs

A T A CAFÉ ON A BUSY ROAD across the street from a hospital, Camilo tells me about his father's bones. The Argentine forensic team identified his father's remains three years ago. He was eighteen months old when his father was disappeared. His mother had been abducted shortly before. The Argentine military targeted young people: Most of those kidnapped and killed were in their twenties, and the children they left behind were usually babies and toddlers. Camilo tells me that after a lifetime of wondering about his father's fate, exhumation and identification have brought him closure: "It closes the story, it ends the grief." Then he leans back and lights a cigarette. A siren passes close by. He inhales, looks up, and says, in a different tone of voice, "Yeah, it's true that it closes things, but in reality, it *opens*. . . . Really, finding mi viejo wasn't the end; it was the beginning. The question is—the beginning of what?"

The beginning of what? Camilo's question sticks with me. Exhumation is often treated as the end of the story. But what if, like Camilo says, it is only the beginning?

The idea that opening graves brings closure for families of the missing makes a lot of sense intuitively. As archaeologist Layla Renshaw writes, exhumation "satisfies the widely held belief that the recovery of human remains is indispensable in order to enact death rituals, enable healthy mourning, and achieve psychological closure." But listening to Camilo and other families and friends of the disappeared convinces me that what exhumation actually does is far more complicated. It ends something, but it also begins. As a poet told me about receiving his father's bones: "Recovering a father disappeared by the dictatorship implies many things, but I never wanted to close anything, actually quite the opposite. For me, it is a process of opening, which still continues."

. . .

CAMILO'S FATHER WAS a guerrilla. Camilo's uncle was a member of the same faction. The brothers were allies, deeply committed to the revolution. Both were disappeared. When the EAAF began the identification process, they suspected they had found one of the brothers. But which one?

In Guatemala, a similar situation arose when the military killed two brothers in a massacre. In the exhumation, the body of one of the brothers was recovered, but traditional forms of forensic identification could not determine which of the two men had been found: There were no distinguishing features like an arm broken in childhood or a chipped tooth. Nor could a DNA analysis settle the matter. Neither brother had children, and with only maternal and paternal genetic samples to analyze, there was no way to tell them apart. This was a source of pain for the family. Who had been found? Science had no answer. Then, their father had a dream. His younger son appeared to him to say that it was his body the forensic team had unearthed. In the archives of the forensic lab, the case file reflects the scientific view that the recovered remains could be those of either brother. But for the family, the case is closed, the dream identification was conclusive, and they held a funeral for the younger brother.

Camilo and his cousin Félix waited for the results of the DNA match. In the end, the remains proved to belong to Camilo's father. He was invited to see his father's bones in the lab, where, as part of the restitution process, a team member would answer his questions and reconstruct the skeleton. Camilo debated. He felt queasy about seeing the bones. But it would be his only chance to see his father's body—when bones are exhumed, they surface from the depths, but not for long. They must be reburied or cremated. The body appears only to quickly disappear again. If he was to see the bones, he had to catch them as they flashed through the world of the living. So Camilo went to the EAAF lab. He didn't really want to go, but he worried that if he didn't, he might someday wish he had. He made a calculation about regret and time and stepped into a small room where his father's bones had been arranged on a table.

Camilo cannot remember his father, "at least not on a conscious level," as he puts it. He peppers his conversation with references to psychology and therapy. This is not unusual in Argentina, a country steeped in psychoanalytic thought. According to the World Health Organization, Argentina has the most psychologists per capita of any country; the runner-up has half the number. While not every psychologist in Argentina is a psychoanalyst, many are. A neighborhood in Buenos Aires is known as "Villa Freud" because it is so densely packed with psychoanalysts' offices. Argentine public hospitals regularly prescribe psychoanalysis in addition to psychiatric medication. Some prisons provide analysis. When the rest of the world abandoned talk therapy in favor of antidepressants and cognitive-behavioral approaches in the 1990s, Argentina staunchly clung to psychoanalysis. References to Sigmund Freud, Jacques Lacan, Melanie Klein, and Alfred Adler aren't limited to therapists' offices or academic conferences; they abound in newspaper columns, television talk shows, podcasts, jokes, and internet memes. Camilo is not an outlier when he tells me, using psychoanalytic terminology, that to grieve and emerge from that grief, "I had to kill the father."

After our conversation, I track down a half-remembered passage in a book: "The work of mourning involves killing the dead. The mourner has the choice of killing the dead or dying with them." It's a text inspired by Freud and the French psychoanalyst Lacan, who reworked many of Freud's foundational concepts. Lacan's books and public lectures are notoriously dense, but his obscurantism sometimes flared with brilliance. A complex and controversial figure, Lacan held therapy sessions for ten minutes or three hours, seduced patients, freely belched and farted, all while rubbing shoulders with the most prominent intellectuals of his day. In Argentina, Lacan has the status of a psychoanalytic rock star. The rapid rise in popularity of Lacanian analysis roughly coincided with the years of the military dictatorship. Some scholars attribute this timing to the complexity of Lacanian language, which Argentine intellectuals utilized as a code they hoped would be impenetrable to the junta's spies and task forces.

Lacan developed his thoughts on "killing the dead" through the Greek tragedy *Antigone*. Its barest outline tells the story of Antigone's two brothers, rulers of Thebes, who cannot share power and go to war. They both die, and their uncle Creon becomes king. He declares one brother, Polynices, a traitor and forbids him to be mourned or buried on pain of death. Grieving her favorite brother, Antigone defies the royal decree. When she's caught, she says that she has a divine right to bury her brother no matter the king's law. As punishment, Creon buries her alive in a cave. He changes his mind and decides to free her, but it is too late; Antigone has already hanged herself.

Antigone is the popular saint of disappearance, invoked in the titles of documentary films and the texts of academic articles, usually offered as a morality tale about the fundamental right to bury the dead. But Greek tragedies are not a genre known for their simplicity and clarity, and Lacan's reading centers Antigone's ethical complexity. Antigone is caught: If she doesn't bury her brother, she faces spiritual death; if she buries him, she faces physical death. As Antigone is suspended between two deaths and literally buried alive in a cave, Lacan says she radiates "unbearable splendor." Her refusal to loosen her bonds to her dead brother—to "kill the dead"—is at once revolutionary and fatal.

There is a trace of Antigone's splendor and tragedy in something the son of a disappeared father told me: that if he could have one thing in life, a single wish fulfilled, he would wish to find his father's body. A father himself, he felt guilty about this desire: "I know I should wish something for my son," he said, "wish for his success." But his deepest desire was to bury his father. The dead father eclipsed the living son.

Camilo grew up worshipful of his revolutionary father. "But that's not the whole story." His father, as Camilo sees it now, was single-minded in his commitment to his cause. He was courageous, but he was also reckless. He had already been detained and tortured once. He must have known he wouldn't be released from a secret prison twice. When Camilo's mother discovered she was pregnant, she wanted to stop living in hiding, but he refused, and they separated. When his friends and comrades were disappeared, Camilo's father continued. "What was going to happen was very predictable," says Camilo. Like Antigone, his father was relentless in his desire. He chose the struggle over everything else. Camilo pauses. "Over me." For Camilo, to symbolically "kill the father" is to dismantle and abandon the heroic figure he had imagined as a child and to recognize, in fragments of stories, photos, and bones, a human being—brave, flawed, mysterious.

. . .

A PSYCHOANALYST WHO works with families of the disappeared told me about mothers who keep their children's rooms untouched and fathers who refuse to move to a new house because what if their children come back and cannot find them? While this may appear to outsiders as denial or even madness, the psychoanalyst had a more subtle diagnosis. She said that even when it was clear that the missing child would not be coming back, even when the family acknowledged this, they would never say of their child, "They are dead." Because to say this would be to symbolically kill them.

Listening to the stories of families, I think that to know a child is lost and yet never declare them dead, to defiantly guard a symbolic space between life and death, takes the rapt concentration and care of defusing a bomb, but goes on for decades.

The parents of disappeared children protect their memories like hands cupped around a match. The children of missing parents work to stir memory's embers, to keep them lit. Both are burdened by heavy symbolic tasks, but distinct ones, as the work of parenting is different from the work of growing up. Leaving families to do this difficult labor—to refuse to symbolically "kill" the child or to be forced to symbolically "kill the father"—is one of the many cruelties of disappearance.

After the abductions, families of the disappeared were often abandoned in their grief. They became marked. Friends, neighbors, and even other family members shunned them. One mother relates: "After my son and his wife disappeared, I never again heard from any of my six sisters or my brother. They all avoided us." People whispered about the disappeared, "They must have done something." People stayed away, afraid they would be seen as fraternizing with subversives and meet the same fate. To shield themselves, people constructed thin shelters of blame, denial, and the "anticipatory obedience" that accompanies tyranny. "Most of the power of authoritarianism is freely given," as historian Timothy Snyder warns. "Individuals think ahead about what a more repressive government will want, and then offer themselves without being asked." Terror travels from a family to their neighbors, to the city, until everyone is afraid and silent. Torture is transmitted from one body to many bodies and finally to the social body of an entire country.

I once spoke to a sympathizer of the military dictatorship. I hadn't realized this about him, but it became clear during our conversation. As he walked me out, I noticed a small, framed sign in the lobby of his apartment building. Faded, hanging in a corner, it read SILENCE IS HEALTH. This infamous motto of the dictatorship was ostensibly part of a campaign to curb urban noise pollution, but everyone understood the subtext: Say nothing, and you may be spared. The hairs on the back of my arms stood up. I wanted to take a photo of the sign as proof I had seen it, but the sympathizer was standing next to me, so I pretended I didn't know what it meant; I kept silent.

. . .

IN A PHOTOGRAPH taken a few months before his disappearance, Camilo's father is at the beach, dangling his baby son in the surf. His father is tan and happy. Baby Camilo smiles. The sun shines. Camilo has a recurring dream about being in the ocean with his father. In the dream, Camilo is older, maybe seven. His father stands in deep water, holding him. Camilo says, "He is teaching me how to swim," and gestures wrapping his hands around a boy's small chest. As he speaks, the mood shifts. An image of father and son shimmers between us, appearing like a photograph developed in a darkroom. Camilo, who is usually frenetic and joking, becomes still. He is visibly shaken and close to tears.

When he speaks again, it is to wonder if the dream is a memory, primordially and wordlessly formed during that long-ago trip to the beach. Or had the images from the dream been etched in his mind from looking a thousand times at the old photo?

Philosopher Roland Barthes calls the ability of a photograph to wound us its "punctum," a term rooted in the Greek word for puncture—capturing how a poignant detail can fly like an arrow from an image and pierce us. Barthes also writes that photographs of the missing beloved touch us "like the delayed rays of a star," a wounding that is also radiant. Like stars, bones are otherworldly—belonging not to outer space but to the underworld and the inner world. Like photographs, bones are strange relics, half material and half spirit.

.　.　.

IN THE EAAF lab, Camilo watched as a forensic anthropologist "put together the human puzzle of my father," articulating the bones in anatomical order. They were the size and shape of a man, but he did not see them as his father. "Of course, I *believed* it was him, but I didn't *feel* it was him."

Bones invite and resist meaning. Writing on violence, the philosopher Achille Mbembé notes of bones "their strange coolness on one hand, and on the other, their stubborn will to mean, to signify something." Camilo was given an urn containing his father's bones. He brought it home and kept it with him for three days. He wanted to feel the presence of his father. He willed the bones to signify something. He even slept with the urn by his side one night. At first, he tells me the story in comic terms. "My girlfriend wouldn't share the bed with me; she thought it was creepy as hell," he says, laughing. But then he says with sadness in his voice, "I wanted to feel something, but I didn't. I kept trying, but it didn't happen."

.　.　.

TO RECOGNIZE A missing person in a bone is a difficult act of imagination. This became clear to me on a rainy winter morning I spent with a woman named Dulce, whose brother had been found in Pozo de Vargas. The forensic team had recovered only a fragment of his pelvis, from which a DNA match had been made. Dulce told me, "It is good to find even a piece of bone. It gives you something to write your grief on." But she was also disturbed by this fragment and said several times, "Is this little thing him?" and "What happened to the rest of him?" Dulce spoke with such immediacy that I began to feel that the bone was present, that it must be somewhere in her small apartment. I knew this was not possible; it would not be allowed. Anyway, Dulce had told me earlier that her family had held a funeral service and buried the bone, following some debate about what was to be done if more pieces were later identified. Still, I found myself searching for the fragment on the windowsill among the seashells and chunks of driftwood, faded white like bones.

The immediacy of Dulce's preoccupation may have been a sign of trauma, with its hallmark disturbances in time in which the terrible event that could not be integrated into experience in the past continues to irrupt, vital, butting into the present. She insisted that finding the fragment had brought her "peace" and "healing," but in the next breath, she said, "It has destroyed me."

"It's a complicated situation. I've had a lot of therapy in my life. I've suffered from melancholy," Dulce told me with such pain in her voice that I stopped the interview early and sat with her, drinking yerba mate and playing cards, not wanting to leave her alone.

One definition of melancholy is finally getting the "desired object" only to find it disappointing. In this sense, exhumation can be nothing other than melancholic: The "desired object" is the missing person—the brother, the daughter, the father—but the "getting," the return, is always only bones. Exhumation never brings back the beloved.

Later, working alongside Santiago in the depths of Pozo de Vargas, I thought of Dulce as I scraped mud from bones. I wondered if the fragment of bone I was touching belonged to her brother, and if it did, would its discovery bring her healing or pain?

. . .

"CLOSURE THROUGH A traditional funeral" is a primary objective of exhumation. In a sense, the whole point of an exhumation is to unearth bodies so they can be buried again, but this time with ritual and a name.

From an anthropological point of view, mourning practices and funeral rites have vast variation. Humans bury and burn our dead, leave our dead to be reclaimed by the elements and eaten by scavengers. We wrap the dead in fabric, cover them in shells, leave them curled in a fetal position or flat on their backs. We dig up the dead and inspect their bones. We keep the dead in houses and under the floors of churches. We mourn by chanting the names of the dead. We grieve by forbidding that the names of the dead be spoken.

In the multitude of mortuary rituals, exhumation has a precise cultural lineage, a genealogy traced to the founding father of psychoanalysis—Sigmund Freud.

Freud's theories, particularly those presented in *Mourning and Melancholia,* published in 1917, have profoundly shaped contemporary conceptions of grief. In this essay, he argues that while mourning is worked through in time, melancholy persists and "behaves like an open wound." In other words, mourning ends, but melancholy is endless. Even as more recent psychological theories expand, amend, contest, or strive to replace the original Freudian model, the idea of grief as a linear and progressive process leading to "closure" stubbornly persists.

. . .

PSYCHOLOGICAL THEORIES OF grief travel with much older beliefs about the care of the dead body. Anthropologists consider funeral rites to be culturally universal. The ritual care of the dead stretches back as far as the beginning of humanity and as wide as humans have settled. Historian Thomas Laqueur says, "We care for the dead because humans have always cared for our dead."

Generations of psychologists have claimed that the absence of a body inevitably renders the grieving process pathologically "complicated," "impeded," or "frozen." Following Freudian thought, psychologists have theorized that encountering the corpse proves to mourners that the death is real, and that this form of "reality testing" is a crucial step in the grief process. Freud believed that the work of mourning involved "decathexis," a withdrawal of psychological energy. This odd word, "cathexis," is a neologism. It is a translation of the very ordinary German word "Besetzung," which has a range of meanings, like "to charge" as with electricity, "to occupy" as with troops or with thoughts, and "to set in place" like a gemstone. The Freudian view holds that when mourners see the corpse, they cut the electric charge, pull back the troops, reclaim the jewel—they clearly understand that their loved one is dead.

Eighty years after Freud's essay on mourning and melancholy, psychologist Pauline Boss introduced the influential theory of "ambiguous loss," arguing that without a body, grief cannot come to "normal closure." Among the many cases she describes are disappearances. She writes, "Consider an old woman in Bosnia hugging a fleshless skull that she takes for her son, on the sketchy evidence of a familiar shoe found nearby. This woman is suffering from a unique kind of loss that defies closure."

The long legacy of Freud's theory of mourning and melancholy shapes how psychologists think about the tragedy of disappearance, particularly in Argentina, a country suffused with psychoanalytic thought. Argentine psychoanalyst Lucia Corti writes that for families of the disappeared, "The absence of the body, and therefore the impossibility of giving burial to the dead, poses a fundamental problem in the mourning process." Or, as psychoanalyst Cecilia Taiana puts it more bluntly: "Survivors of the disappeared face endless melancholia."

This psychological heritage has also shaped forensic exhumation, evident in the promise that recovering the bodies of the missing brings mourners closure. A report from the International Committee of the Red Cross states that for families of the missing, the absence of a body "prevents them from mourning properly." According to Interpol, identification of remains provides the "opportunity to mourn and achieve closure." Yet a difficult truth of exhumation is that many bodies will never be found. That is the cruel logic of disappearance. Many sites of violence will never be located or investigated due to a lack of political will and a paucity of funding. Even when clandestine graves are excavated, not all remains will be identified.

Most families of the missing will never have a body to mourn or bury. Does this mean they are condemned to bear their grief as an open wound? Even for those families who recover bodies, if "reality testing" depends on recognizing that the beloved is dead, what does this mean for those who receive only a single bone? For those who cannot recognize their beloved in a fragment? How does the presence of the body help mourning when a piece of pelvis is all that remains of a brother? When a skeleton is nothing like a father?

Josefina, an elegant woman with a warm and intelligent gaze, told me about her complex experience of identification and return. Her father, Dardo Francisco Molina, an eminent politician, Perónist, and vice-governor of the province of Tucumán, was disappeared during the dictatorship. One of his teeth was found in the Pozo de Vargas and matched by DNA. A year later, part of his hip was identified. A year after that, his femur. Then his blood-stained clothing. And so it went, meter by meter, piece by piece—vertebrae, scapula, ribs—her father was returned to her. She says that she planted a tree when she received her father's tooth. But what was she to do as each fragment surfaced? How could she make sense of "seven griefs"? His complete skeleton has never been recovered. She tells me that this, too, is one of the cruelties of the junta.

. . .

THE LAST NIGHT that Camilo had his father's bones in his possession, family and friends gathered for an intimate memorial. A classmate from high school brought a forgotten home movie, on old Super 8 mm film unearthed from a closet. The short clip showed Camilo's father at a backyard asado, barbecuing and joking around. Camilo watched the clip over and over. He was mesmerized by the swing of his father's arms, how he turned his head, how he squinted. It was the first time Camilo had seen his father in motion other than in dreams.

It was only by chance that Camilo saw the film in the presence of the bones, but their meeting gave rise to a tension, a disjuncture in time. The movie was from the past—the bones were in the present. The body in the film was alive and moving—Camilo recognized his father. The body in the urn was unmoving and lifeless—Camilo could not recognize his father. Which was more his father, the flicker of light on the screen or the bones in the urn?

When everyone had gone home, Camilo sat alone on the edge of his bed next to the urn of bones. He felt a sense of urgency. Tomorrow morning, the bones would be gone. There was little time. And then, it happened. Camilo tells me that suddenly "he was real." Camilo curled his body around the urn and "cried like a baby all night."

• • •

CAMILO'S ENCOUNTER WITH his father's bones doesn't fit neatly into theories of grief and mourning. He had recovered his father's remains, but the bones didn't invite "reality testing" and "decathexis" in Freud's sense. Reality testing says, "I can't believe it is him; it can't be him." But Camilo was doing the opposite, willing himself to believe it was his father in front of him, insisting "it must be him." Contrary to severing ties and withdrawing energy, Camilo was trying hard to charge his father's bones with meaning, to occupy their cool presence with love. In many family members of the disappeared, I witnessed the imaginative work seeking to connect memories, dreams, a box of bones, DNA results, old letters, photos, film clips—everything at hand—to trace the shape of the beloved.

• • •

SEVERAL MONTHS LATER, Camilo and I meet again. We sit at a sidewalk café and drink orange sodas as the heat of the day softens. He is eager to talk. He says, "I have to tell you about this thing that happened since I saw you last." He pauses. "We had a funeral for my uncle."

"Where did they find his body?"

"Well, they didn't find it, not exactly."

A few months earlier, Camilo's cousin Félix had surprised the family by saying that he wanted to organize a funeral for his father, body or no body. He had already started making the arrangements at Chacarita Cemetery in Buenos Aires. The way Félix saw it, his father had probably been killed in a death flight, and his body would probably never be recovered. Since there was no hope that his father's remains would be found, he didn't want to wait any longer to have a funeral and the chance to say goodbye.

Félix tells me that going through the experience with Camilo made him think. "It was galvanizing, it kind of reopened things . . . wounds and questions that are buried in your mind." It started at the EAAF lab, when he saw his uncle's bones "very lovingly presented" on a beautiful piece of Latin American fabric. He says, "It brought me peace. I arrived feeling upset and I left feeling at peace."

Afterward, he thought about how even though he was certain his father was dead, he had never had a ceremony to say goodbye. "I embarked on a process to understand this thing happening to me and to give it form." He started to read about funeral rites. "For the Greeks, children had one obligation to their parents. Only one, which was to arrange their funeral." He read about the pyramids, the Tomb of the Unknown Soldier, and how Romans cremated their dead. He researched cenotaphs—monuments to honor the dead without the body present; the term comes from the Greek words for "empty" and "tomb." He thought about how there have always been people who died and whose bodies have gone missing. Sailors and fishermen lost at sea. Mountain climbers and hunters who never return from the forest. Victims of plane crashes. "In the history of humanity it is much more common to have a ceremony without a body than to have someone die—be disappeared—without a ceremony."

"If he's disappeared, then he could appear again, right?" Félix's young son asked him one day. They were the words of a child who had never been exposed to the perverse language of the dictatorship, who didn't know General Videla's speech: "The disappeared are just that: disappeared; they are neither alive nor dead; they are disappeared." His son's question impacted him. A funeral ritual would offer an essential affirmation that his father wasn't missing, he had been murdered. His *body* was disappeared, but *he* was dead. "A symbolic change of status, in a sense," Félix tells me. He chose Chacarita because it is a legendary cemetery; in tango songs and Buenos Aires slang, "to go to Chacarita" means to die, like English speakers might say "to kick the bucket." A monument in Chacarita was a way to publicly acknowledge his father's death.

. . .

"APARICIÓN CON VIDA" is one of the Madres' best-known slogans, and one of the most difficult, divisive, and mysterious. It literally demands "appearance with life" in the face of disappearance. It has been interpreted in religious terms, as a political strategy, as a sign of trauma or denial, and as a kind of koan— a riddle without a solution that reveals a deeper truth. "Aparición con vida" is a slogan used to reject exhumation. It highlights how fraught symbolic change of a status between disappearance and death can be.

. . .

NOT ALL FAMILIES of the missing want exhumations, a truth which isn't always widely acknowledged in forensic circles. Families in Cyprus and Spain have opposed exhumations. Jewish communities in Poland have organized resistance to the excavation of Holocaust mass graves, citing religious laws forbidding disturbing the dead. The family of poet Federico García Lorca, who was disappeared during the Spanish Civil War, publicly disputed a proposal to exhume his body from a suspected mass grave, writing, "We would choose to leave Lorca where he is, in the company of all victims." The wishes of Lorca's family were overruled, and the suspected mass grave was exhumed with much media attention. In the end, no bodies were found at the site.

In 1985, at an early exhumation, the EAAF arrived at a grave only to be greeted by about fifteen women, yelling and throwing stones. It was the Madres de Plaza de Mayo. The young team reacted with disbelief and shock, imagining themselves as allies. "It was hard to see that these women, who were our heroes, were against us," said Mimi Doretti. They left the exhumation site and went to a beach near the cemetery. "We sat there, looking at the ocean, shattered."

Some Madres saw exhumations as a surreptitious attempt to convert mass atrocity into private grief. Hebe de Bonafini, who protested the exhumation that day, puts it this way: "Many want the wound to dry so that we will forget. We want it to continue bleeding." Such a stance rejects "closure" in favor of the wound left purposefully open—a willful political melancholia.

In 1986, the Madres split into two groups, partly over disagreements about exhumations. One group, "Madres de Plaza de Mayo Línea Fundadora," supports them. The other group, "Asociación Madres de Plaza de Mayo," headed by Hebe de Bonafini, adamantly rejects them.

. . .

BETWEEN MOTHERS OF the disappeared there are conflicting views. Within one family, opinions proliferate, experiences differ, and approaches diverge. "Grieving breaks us apart, indeed, and keeps us together," as writer Cristina Rivera Garza observes, reckoning with the losses wrought by violence in her own country, Mexico.

In Spain, construction workers expanding a road found human remains and a suspected mass grave from the country's civil war. Believing his father to be among the dead, Antonio de León appealed to the mayor to excavate. But his brother, Fernando de León, was not in agreement, and petitioned a judge to block the exhumation. The two brothers feuded over whether their father's body should be recovered or left where it was buried.

In Argentina, when the remains of Jorge Daniel Argente were identified by the EAAF, his family couldn't agree on what kind of funeral they wanted. Daniel's brother Hugo relates that their sister suggested a small, private ceremony. He vehemently rejected the idea: "This is a thing that the whole world has to know about, that a person who has been missing for twenty-four years was murdered by the military." They buried Daniel in Chacarita with five hundred people in attendance. Hugo says, "That ritual, that burial, was a denunciation, rather than something that helped me in my grieving; otherwise I would have had to do something intimate like my sister said. It was a political act."

A brother finds meaning in gathering a crowd at Chacarita to say "Never Again." A sister finds meaning in quietly placing flowers on a grave. Some families are comforted by a funeral mass and a marble angel in a cemetery. Some seek out the angel of history, facing the wreckage of the past, the catastrophe that cannot be reconciled, as Walter Benjamin wrote.

. . .

WHILE *MOURNING AND MELANCHOLIA* was Freud's most influential work on grief, it does not represent his final thoughts on the subject. In later years, he substantially revised his theories. Reflecting on his original views, he wrote that he had not at first appreciated the significance of melancholy, how common it is, and how it makes an "essential contribution" toward building the "character" of the ego. Rather than see melancholy as a pathology, Freud came to see it as a deeply human process, indeed the process that makes us human. Losses leave traces, and it is from these fragments that we construct ourselves as mature human beings—aware of fragility, interdependent with others. As lines from a poem by Jorge Luis Borges say:

We are our memory
we are that chimerical museum of shifting shapes
that pile of broken mirrors.

In part, Freud's revisions came through his own experiences of grief. In 1920, his daughter Sophie, whom he adored and called his "Sunday Child," died of the flu. Her death came at the end of the pandemic, when the danger seemed to have passed. Her young son died three years later. These losses affected Freud deeply. Nine years after Sophie's death, Freud wrote to a friend whose son had recently died. He offered his condolences and said:

"We know that the acute sorrow we feel after such a loss will run its course, but also that we will remain inconsolable, and will never find a substitute. No matter what may come to take its place, even should it fill that place completely, it remains something else. And that is how it should be." Grief persists, in its complexity and mystery, as "something else"—for a long time, maybe forever. And that is how it should be. In Freud's later work, the lost beloved is not "replaced" so much as "re-placed," as psychoanalyst Salman Akhtar observes. He writes that in grief, the dead are "psychically relocated," an insight with particular poignancy for exhumation, in which families must also physically relocate the dead.

Like Freud, psychologist Pauline Boss also altered her theories of mourning. The year after she published her influential book on ambiguous loss, she began working with families of people killed in the 2001 attacks on the World Trade Center in New York. She came to call closure "a myth." She found that families of the missing could grieve in ways that were healthy and that most found resolution not through closure but in meaning making. Fredy Peccerelli, director of the Guatemalan team, has also evolved in his understanding. "I used to think exhumations brought closure," he said. "Now I think they bring empowerment."

Recent psychological research on grief favors meaning making over closure; accepts zigzagging paths, not just linear stages;

recognizes ambiguity without pathology; and acknowledges continuing bonds between the living and the dead rather than commanding decathexis. But old ideas about grief as a linear march to closure still hold powerful sway. Many psychologists and grief counseling programs continue to consider "closure" a therapeutic goal. Sympathy cards, internet searches, and friendly advice often uphold a rigid division between healthy grief that the mourner "gets over" and unhealthy grief that persists. Forensic exhumation, too, continues to be informed by these deeply rooted ideas.

The experiences of grief and exhumation related by families of the missing indicate something more complex and mysterious than "closure." Exhumation heals and wounds, sometimes both at once, in the same gesture, in the same breath, as Dulce described feeling consoled and destroyed by the fragment of her brother's bones. Exhumation can divide brothers and restore fathers, open old wounds and open the possibility of regeneration—of building something new with the "pile of broken mirrors" that is memory, loss, and mourning.

CHAPTER 11

Southern Cross

I MEET ANA MARÍA CAREAGA in the urban neighborhood of San Cristóbal on the corner of Urquiza and Estados Unidos streets. The air is milky and bright after days of rain. Iglesia Santa Cruz is still closed for renovation, but a priest has agreed to give us a tour. The exterior of the church is wrapped in scaffolding, and a few flanks of clean pink stone show through. It was built in the nineteenth century for Irish immigrants, masses were held in English until the 1930s, and it is still sometimes referred to as the "Irish church" in the neighborhood.

Father Carlos Saracini meets us on the front steps. He is openfaced and smiling. He's wearing jeans and a wooden cross and greets us warmly, locking his intense green eyes on me. He embraces Ana María, and I realize they know each other well. Ana María introduces me, saying, "I was just telling her what a character you are. Like out of a movie!" He laughs. "But which movie? That makes all the difference!"

. . .

IN ARGENTINA, THE question "Which Catholicism?" made all the difference during the dictatorship. The junta was allied with the church from the start. In early footage of the coup, bishops flank the military leaders, their red hats and sashes flashing in a sea of military uniforms. Yet, while the church and armed forces had what one historian calls a relationship of "symbiosis," El Proceso also targeted priests and nuns for disappearance. In a country that was 90 percent Catholic, in most cases the torturers and their victims shared the same religion, though they understood its teachings in diametrically different terms.

. . .

FATHER CARLOS OPENS the door to the sanctuary. It is cool and dark. The wood floors are clean and worn. Because it is still under renovation and closed to the public, it feels like a secret place. He turns on the lights from a breaker box, illuminating the soaring ceiling, marble arches, and stained-glass windows made in Dublin, their brilliance muted by the scaffolding and the cocoon of plastic sheeting outside. The pews have been arranged into circles "to break up the hierarchy," Father Carlos explains.

. . .

CHURCH AND STATE had long been closely linked in Argentina, a land of "the cross and the sword." The state even paid the salaries of Catholic priests. But in the years leading up to the junta, priests and nuns across Latin America began forging new forms of religious practice rooted in social justice, like liberation theology and Argentina's homegrown "Third World Priest Movement." They left their cloisters to work and live among the poor.

In many places, the church openly defied right-wing dictators. In Guatemala, Bishop Juan José Gerardi led a truth commission to uncover the human rights abuses of La Violencia. In Chile, Archbishop Raúl Silva Henríquez spoke out against the Pinochet dictatorship. In El Salvador, Bishop Oscar Romero publicly decried the military's atrocities.

In Argentina, by contrast, the Catholic hierarchy demonstrated "decisive overwhelming support" for the dictatorship. One archbishop publicly welcomed the coup, giving a sermon in which he mused: "Will Christ not wish someday for the armed forces to go beyond their usual function?"

High-ranking members of the clergy were close to the junta, serving as advisers, confessors, and friends. Admiral Emilio Eduardo Massera, the navy's representative in the junta, regularly played tennis with nuncio Pio Laghi, the pope's ambassador in Argentina. General Jorge Rafael Videla was personal friends with Monsignor Adolfo Tortolo. In media interviews shortly before his death, Videla said that the junta's relationship with the church was "excellent, very cordial, sincere, and open." He said that the junta kept church officials apprised of disappearances, and "they advised us on how to handle it."

. . .

ANA MARÍA AND Father Carlos are proud of the church and excited to show me details. They point out the hand-lettered signs on the walls, white sheets spray-painted with messages of solidarity like PASSION FOR JUSTICE, TRUTH, AND LOVE, a reference to the church's order, the Pasionistas, whose motto is "In solidarity with the crucified of today."

"Who are the crucified of today?" I ask Father Carlos. He responds, "The poor, people living in villas miserias, Indigenous communities struggling for their lands."

We spend a long time looking at a painting by Adolfo Pérez Esquivel, an artist and activist. He won the Nobel Peace Prize in 1980 for his human rights work in Argentina, advocacy for which he was also detained and tortured in a secret prison for more than a year. The work is part of a series Pérez Esquivel created to commemorate five hundred years of the conquest of the Americas (1492–1992). *El Paño de Cuaresma,* also known as *Resurrected Jesus with a Latin American Face Walking with His People,* depicts a skinny, brown-skinned, barefoot messiah surrounded by a triumphant crowd. Ana María and Father Carlos point out figures on the canvas. Here is Pachamama, Mother Earth, growing maize. Here is Chico Mendes, who fought for workers and the rain forest. Here is Zumbi dos Palmares, who led an uprising against slavery in Brazil. Here is the Inca revolutionary Túpac Amaru. Here are the Madres in their white headscarves.

Father Carlos shows me a glass case near the altar with two relics, one from Saint Paul of the Cross, who founded the Pasionistas in the eighteenth century. The other is a small scrap of fabric.

"What is it?" I ask.

Father Carlos says, "This is from the great martyr, Father Mugica." It is a piece of the shirt he was wearing when murdered. Carlos Mugica, who is depicted among the crowd in the painting, was a priest from a wealthy Argentine family who dedicated himself to working with the poor. He was influential in the Catholic youth movement of the 1960s. Several of his students founded the Montoneros, a group he first supported and later distanced himself from but never cut ties with. His sermons, delivered at Christ the Worker chapel in Villa 31, became enormously popular. After giving a sermon on May 11, 1974, he was assassinated by an agent of the Triple A death squad, controlled by El Brujo. Argentina's most outspoken priest was murdered before the junta even began.

This was the fate of those in the church who challenged the military leaders and the ultraconservative Catholicism they sanctioned. Bishop Enrique Ángel Angelelli Carletti, who is also pictured in the painting, was run off the road in La Rioja Province in what the military tried to frame as a car crash. Angelelli had predicted his assassination, knowing that his work for a "Church of the Poor" made him a target. In the city of Córdoba, a group of six priests and seminary students were abducted and imprisoned at the secret detention center La Perla.

And, of course, there is the case of Sister Alice Domon, abducted from the church where we are standing. She was taken with Ana María's mother, Esther, and the other Madres, followed soon afterward by Sister Léonie Duquet. The two French nuns look out from Pérez Esquivel's painting, and a large banner with their photos hangs by the altar. Sister Alice and Sister Léonie worked together teaching at a school for disabled children, where one of their students was General Videla's son Alejandro. Sister Alice lived in Villa 20 in Buenos Aires. Her friends and neighbors, many of them immigrants from Bolivia and Paraguay, remembered her buoyant spirit: how she tried to tell jokes before she could even speak Spanish, disappointed when no one laughed along with her. Later she moved to the rural province of Corrientes, where she helped tobacco workers organize for better working conditions. As the political climate became increasingly authoritarian, several tobacco workers were disappeared. The nuns she was working with suspended the project, deeming it too dangerous. Sister Alice objected. Frustrated by their lack of commitment, she returned to the city to work with the Madres.

Sister Alice understood the risk. In September 1976, she wrote a letter saying: "The persecution grows worse, I don't know where it will all end.... You may have heard about what has happened to other priests and nuns. I wouldn't say it makes me feel anxious. In fact, I feel very calm because I know that I'm on the right path and it's a cause worth dying for." In Buenos Aires, she moved into a safe house. In her last letter to her family in France, dated November 8, 1977, a month before she was abducted, she wrote about her work with the mothers of the disappeared: "It is interesting that suffering can enable people to grow as much as it can also destroy them. Our prayer must extend to all and be expressed in different forms, like a hunger strike, a political rally, a letter to the bishops, etc.... We must regret nothing. We must forge ahead."

During the dictatorship, the most dangerous act for priests and nuns was working with the poor, which the junta interpreted as a sign of Marxist infiltration of the church. A priest held in the infamous La Perla camp testified that his torturers called him "an angel with black wings" for his work in villas miserias. They said, "It's worse that you work with the poor because when you work with them, the poor feel encouraged, they join together and become dangerous." A guard at ESMA told Father Orlando Yorio, "You are not a guerrilla fighter. You are not in the violence." The reason for his torture and imprisonment was "you unite the poor and uniting the poor is subversion." Another priest held at La Perla was interrogated by a torturer who went by the nickname "the Priest." The false priest lectured the real priest in theological doctrine, saying that the rich were rich and the poor were poor according to God's will, and to change that was subversive.

Iglesia Santa Cruz was one of the few parishes that publicly resisted the junta. In their weekly paper, *The Southern Cross,* they directly criticized the church's role in the dictatorship in editorials such as "The Silence of the Bishops." They opened their doors to the Madres and sheltered political refugees from other parts of Latin America. They lodged the Permanent Assembly for Human Rights, which included Catholic priests, activists like Pérez Esquivel and lawyer Emilio Mignone, as well as Protestant and Jewish leaders. The group's documentation of human rights abuses later made foundational contributions to the truth commission report. Santa Cruz was a refuge for human rights activists and dissidents—until it became a site of betrayal and death.

Five priests and seminary students were executed at Saint Patrick's Church, an Irish congregation in the suburbs of Buenos Aires. When the priests at Iglesia Santa Cruz heard about the Saint Patrick's Church massacre, they wondered if the military had made a mistake and meant to target them, a much more politically active Irish church. The assassins had left a message scrawled by the bodies of the priests and students: "These lefties died for being brainwashers of innocent minds and members of MSTM," the Spanish acronym for the Third World Priest Movement. In one of their hallucinatory sleights of hand, the army issued a statement after the massacre blaming the atrocities on guerrillas. "Subversive elements cowardly murdered the priests and seminarians," it read, "which shows that the perpetrators, besides having no fatherland, also have no God."

. . .

"EL CURA" WAS a popular nom de guerre for torturers. One "priest" said to his victims before his torments, "Come, my child, give me your confession." But it wasn't just a matter of nicknames and charades; real priests visited secret detention centers, and some extorted confessions during torture. The trial of Christian Federico Von Wernich, the first priest prosecuted for human rights violations during the dictatorship, brought the complicity of the church in the atrocities of the Argentine junta to international attention. A police chaplain, Von Wernich worked in multiple clandestine detention centers, where prisoners remember him saying things like "God wants to know where your friends are" during torture sessions. A prisoner testified, "The worst torture I suffered was from this man, because it was moral torture." He did not confine himself to moral torture. One witness saw Von Wernich at a sink, washing blood off his hands.

Von Wernich offered spiritual succor to perpetrators. An officer described how he watched a military physician inject a group of prisoners directly in the heart with a fatal substance. Afterward, he was given the task of moving their dead bodies. He testified, "Father Von Wernich saw that what had happened had shocked me and spoke to me, telling me that what we had done was necessary; it was a patriotic act and God knew it was for the good of the country." Religious reassurance and moral legitimation of torture by priests was common practice. An admiral said, "When we had doubts, we went to our spiritual advisors, and they put our minds at ease." Priests and chaplains reassured torturers and executioners that God was on their side.

In October 2007, Von Wernich was found guilty for his involvement in seven murders, thirty-one cases of torture, and forty-two kidnappings. He listened to the verdict wearing his priest's collar. The church did not excommunicate him. Behind bars, he continued to serve as a priest, officiating mass for inmates.

. . .

DURING THE BLOOD-SOAKED years of the dictatorship, Jorge Bergoglio, who as a young priest had become friends with Ana María's mother, and who later became Pope Francis, led the Argentine Jesuits. It was a powerful position, and scholars, journalists, and even Hollywood have speculated about his loyalties and actions. Some human rights activists contend that Bergoglio participated in a conspiracy of silence. Some accuse him of active collaboration with the military. Others claim he acted with quiet resistance, working behind the scenes to release prisoners, shelter people, and help those in danger escape the country.

The central focus has been on the kidnapping, detention, and torture of two priests in his order, Orlando Yorio and Franz Jalics. The priests were seized from a villa miseria in Bajo Flores where they were holding a mass. After five months of captivity, Yorio and Jalics were drugged and loaded onto a helicopter—but this was not a death flight. The two men were dumped alive on the outskirts of the city. Father Yorio described their release in his testimony to Argentina's truth commission: "I realized I was in an open field and then plucked up courage and took off my blindfold. I saw the stars."

In a second case, the father of a disappeared woman sought out Bergoglio for help locating his daughter, Elena de la Cuadra, who was five months pregnant at the time of her abduction. According to the family's legal testimony, Bergoglio provided a handwritten letter of introduction to a bishop with connections to the military. The bishop told the family that Elena had given birth to a girl. He said that the baby had been placed with "a good family," and nothing could be done. Elena was never seen again. The family contends that this contradicts Bergoglio's claim that he knew nothing about the military's illegal adoptions until after the dictatorship.

Estela de Carlotto, leader of the Abuelas de Plaza de Mayo, the organization formed to search for stolen babies, claimed that Bergoglio "knew what was happening but didn't do anything." She adds, "We don't think he's a criminal, but he's complicit by omission." Adolfo Pérez Esquivel said, "Perhaps he didn't have the courage of other priests, but he never collaborated with the dictatorship." Father Yorio died in 2000, but Father Jalics went on record in 2013 to say that while he once thought otherwise, after many conversations and much reflection, he had come to believe that "Orlando Yorio and I were not denounced by Father Bergoglio." He also stated, "I am reconciled with what happened and, for my part, I consider it closed."

Many people in Argentina are not reconciled and do not consider it closed. The full extent of the church's involvement in the dictatorship is still coming to light.

. . .

ANA MARÍA TELLS us that she and her sister Mabel will meet with Pope Francis in a few weeks, when he visits Paraguay. She acknowledges that Jorge Bergoglio is a complicated figure for Argentines, but overall, she thinks that he is steering the church in a good direction in his role as pope. "When I hear him speak today about the poor, the excluded, about everybody's right to work and a roof over their heads," she says, "I hear my mother's influence."

A few weeks after our meeting at Santa Cruz, I read about Ana María's visit with Pope Francis in the newspapers. She gave him an old photo of Esther and her team at the lab, among them a young Jorge Bergoglio. "Oh, it's me!" said the pope. He spoke warmly of Esther, telling Ana María and her sister Mabel, "She's the person who taught me to think."

. . .

ANA MARÍA AND Father Carlos show me a banner of the twelve disappeared and tell me their plans to make a better one, with bigger photos that they will frame on the wall. I search for Ana María's mother. The grainy image shows Esther with a reserved expression. In another photo, Azucena smiles broadly. They both look entirely ordinary, with no outward trace of their bravery. There is something striking in the mundanity of the pictures. As if this, too, is the Madres showing us that revolutionary courage can be hidden anywhere: in a chemistry lab, in bedsheets wrapped around broomsticks, tucked into balls of yarn, in an ordinary life.

Pointing to an angel on the ceiling, Father Carlos says, "I'd like to paint over it." Jabbing a finger toward the angel, he says, "It gives the wrong idea. People think that heaven is up there, but it is here—" he gestures to the space between us.

Ana María says, "Let's give her a surprise," with a conspiratorial wink at Father Carlos. He leads us to a door and up a narrow staircase. This is the "bonus track" of the tour, says Ana María, as we climb to the rafters, so high that we are almost close enough to touch the angel on the ceiling. Father Carlos jokingly gestures as if he's throwing a can of paint over it, and Ana María cracks up, making us all laugh more. We climb out on a narrow ledge above the pulpit with a sense of adventure. "Hang on!" says Ana María.

Looking out with a vertiginous view of the sanctuary, Father Carlos says that the Celts designed churches to look like forests and that you can feel the wildness here when the lights are low and the pillars and arches throw their shadows. As if he's invoked it, I sense that force. I suddenly feel like I might start crying. I'm not Catholic or even religious, but something tender and holy has settled around us. Father Carlos reads aloud the words on one of the painted signs on the back wall and then begins to sing them in a beautiful, powerful voice.

In the forest of the sanctuary and the echoing words, I suddenly realize that I've lost my faith. A faith that I did not know I had until it was gone—my faith in humanity. I no longer have the instinctual feeling that people are good. The mass graves are proof that this is not so.

There is no one I can talk to about what I've seen. Not my family or my friends; I want to protect them. Not Santiago at the Pozo or Adriana and Emilia in the lab: They have built the walls necessary to do their work. I think of how Alvaro told me, more than a year ago now, "We have to distance ourselves—not dehumanize, but distance." I have not been able to do this. I am riddled with numbness and sadness. I feel like I could tell Father Carlos about the bones and the ghosts. About the sorrow that has lived in me for months, and how it touches an older sorrow that has lived in me forever. Maybe it is not mine at all, but wells up from the ground of being human, like the spring near my dad's house bubbled up from nowhere by some rocks in a field, connected invisibly to the depths. Maybe like this we are connected to five hundred years of conquest, to the histories of violence we inherit and then perpetuate.

Ana María hugs my shoulder. She has been subjected to the worst of humanity, but nothing has drawn a curtain over the light she radiates. Father Carlos sings to us: "Memory of the joys inviting us to rejoice, memory of the pain calling us to heal, memory of the dreams pushing us to move forward, memory of the blood that tells us—never again." My fieldwork has brought me close to human evil, which has left a mark and caused a wound. But it has also brought me close to courage and solidarity, to people like Ana María and Father Carlos, and to the memory of Esther and Sister Alice. To the teams and their relentless labor, to the families and their grief and resistance. As the words of the song echo and fade, I think about how the root of the word "bless" means "to mark with blood."

. . .

OUR FINAL STOP is the garden. This is where the Madres last met, and it is where Ana María's mother is now buried, among the trees and flower beds.

In late December 1977, bodies washed up on the shores of the beach town of Santa Teresita on the Atlantic Coast, south of Buenos Aires. News reports in France claimed they belonged to the French nuns and the Madres. Declassified documents reveal that at the time, U.S. diplomats also believed these to be the remains of those abducted from Santa Cruz. No investigation was pursued. The bodies were buried unnamed in the General Lavalle Cemetery, where they stayed for twenty-eight years.

In 2005, the EAAF exhumed a section of the cemetery. In tomb twenty-three, they found bones identified as belonging to Esther Ballestrino de Careaga. They identified five sets of skeletal remains in total, all bearing the distinctive trauma patterns of death flights. The others were identified as Azucena Villaflor de De Vincenti, María Ponce de Bianco, Angela Auad, and Sister Léonie Duquet.

Very few bodies have been recovered from death flights. That their bodies appeared on a beach together is remarkable. In a memorial tribute, their children wrote: "These mothers, tireless fighters who gave their lives for their children, could not defeat death, but they were so stubborn that they could defeat oblivion. And they came back. They returned with the sea, as if they had wanted to give account, once again, of that tenacity that characterized them in life. The presence of their remains testifies to what cannot be made to disappear."

For years, Ana María hoped that her mother might have survived. In testimony she presented in Washington, D.C., in September 1979, she said, "A little while ago we received news from Argentina that she is alive." She told the committee, "Sometimes I lose hope of ever seeing her again, but other times I think those hopes help me endure the sorrow." When Ana María spoke to Congress, U.S. officials had been in possession of intelligence about the grim fate of Esther and the others abducted from Iglesia Santa Cruz for nearly two years. Yet it took more than a quarter century for the families to learn the truth and recover the bodies. Standing in the garden, Ana María says, "Hope is the last thing you lose."

The stone markers, low and black, stand in a semicircle. We gather beside the one bearing Esther's name. Ana María tells me they wanted to bury her here at Santa Cruz because it was the "last free ground she ever knew."

It is late in the afternoon and getting cold when we turn away from the graves. There is one more thing Ana María and Father Carlos want me to see, a small sculpture in an alcove by the garden, a pregnant, barefoot girl—a young and vulnerable Mother Mary. They tell me that sometimes they tie a white kerchief on her head, like the Madres, and take her into the streets, into the neighborhood.

I picture sixteen-year-old Ana María caressing her belly and singing to her baby in her prison cell. I think of the Madres betrayed with a kiss. I think of the twelve disappeared and the five returned by the sea. The thousands who will never be found. Those who keep searching and fighting. Those who keep the faith that we can still find heavens between us.

CHAPTER 12

Odysseus

A TRANSPORTATION STRIKE delays shipments to the lab. The bones we have been planning to work on have not arrived. It is Friday afternoon. It doesn't make sense to start a new project, so Emilia, Adriana, and I unexpectedly find ourselves with a few free hours. We use the time to study differences between pre-, post-, and perimortem trauma. Emilia and Adriana have impressive recall of cases and bring out boxes from storage with examples to illustrate various traumas. We feel for smooth borders and rough edges. We study patterns of fractures. As we are wrapping up, they decide to bring out one last box. I can tell there is something significant in store because they both get uncharacteristically quiet and serious.

They take the box into an exam room with a single table. It isn't a room that we ordinarily use. This is where the team brings the families who come to see remains. Emilia begins to efficiently articulate a skeleton. It is immediately apparent that the body has sustained massive trauma on a scale I have never seen. I understand before I am told that this is the body of someone killed in a death flight.

．　．　．

IN 1994, A man approached well-known investigative journalist Horacio Verbitsky as he waited for a subway train in Buenos Aires. The man said he had something to tell him about the dictatorship. On the crowded platform, Verbitsky took him for a survivor of the clandestine prisons and expressed sympathy for what he had been through. "*No, you don't understand*," said the man. He wasn't a victim; he was a perpetrator.

Retired navy officer Adolfo Scilingo described his participation in death flights in a series of interviews recorded over months. He told Verbitsky that prisoners were taken to a room in the basement of ESMA, where they were told they were being "transferred" to a prison in Patagonia. They were told they would be given a "vaccination" before a navy doctor injected them with a powerful sedative and soldiers dragged them onto a plane. On the flight, the doctor injected the victims again before shutting himself in the cockpit, "something to do with the Hippocratic Oath," said Scilingo. He described the pile of clothes left behind in the plane on the flight back to the base.

In three flights, Scilingo pushed prisoners, drugged but alive, into the ocean to their deaths. Once, he lost his footing and was saved by the other soldiers, who grabbed him before he met the same fate as the prisoners. This moment haunted him. He incessantly dreamed of it. Perhaps this slip led him to be the first member of the military to publicly admit to the atrocities of the dictatorship.

Scilingo confessed to killing thirty people. He revealed that death flights took place every Wednesday. According to his account, all officers were required to participate so that everyone was implicated; it was a blood pact. He described the death flights as a "kind of communion." When he had a moment of doubt, a military chaplain assured him it was a "Christian death" because the victims "didn't suffer."

When his confession went public—in newspapers, on television, in a book—it shook the country. After a surge of reckoning in the first days of democracy, Argentina had passed a series of amnesty measures. The landmark convictions of "Argentina's Nuremberg" trial were reversed. The Full Stop law, in 1986, and the Law of Due Obedience, in 1987, protected the military from prosecution and allowed Alfredo Astiz and others who had committed atrocities to live in freedom. In 1990, then-president Carlos Menem pardoned General Jorge Rafael Videla and the other junta leaders. Argentina had drifted into denialism or at least amnesia. Scilingo's admission prompted a confrontation with the violence of the past and national soul-searching.

. . .

DEATH FLIGHTS RESULT in patterns of skeletal trauma that share features with other high-velocity impacts like falls from buildings and bridges. In falls, trauma is determined by height: Greater heights result in greater distribution and severity of fractures on impact. Other significant factors include impact surface, as energy dissipation differs between displaceable mediums, like water, and nondisplaceable mediums, like concrete. Body orientation plays a role, with different landing positions resulting in different patterns of fractures. Horizontal or prone positions, as opposed to "feet first" landings, tend to result in more grievous trauma. The presence of clothing, environmental conditions such as smooth or choppy water, and muscle tension or laxity as influenced by intoxication—in the case of death flights, injection with Pentothal—also affect trauma. Due to the height from which the people were thrown into the Río de la Plata and the Atlantic Ocean, all victims of death flights would have suffered massive skeletal blunt force trauma impossible to survive.

A hot wave of nausea washes over me as I look at the skeleton. I suddenly find myself two steps away from the exam table, recoiled against the wall of the tiny room. I'm holding my hands around my neck in an unconscious defensive posture. The violence is staggering.

We stand in silence looking at the bones. After a long time,

Emilia lifts the cranium to examine the fracture pattern. Adriana studies the mandible and teeth. I approach the table and look at the left femur. This man was alive when he hit the water. Examining his skeleton, I think about the once-living bone. Nourished by veins and capillaries, his bones were absorbing minerals and remodeling; they were flexible and resilient. They were encased by muscle and skin, and anchored by ligaments and tendons. Despite the force of impact, his skeleton remained intact. He is shattered yet whole, like crazing in the glaze of old ceramics.

Forensic anthropology has taught me a radically new way of meeting another human being—not through their biography but through their embodied life history. I decode the messages of trauma written in his skeleton. With nothing more than bones to go on, alphabets of injury can be deciphered to tell a story.

Violence is notoriously difficult to talk about. What words can describe torture? What phrases can explain suffering? In her foundational book *The Body in Pain*, Elaine Scarry writes, "Physical pain does not simply resist language but actively destroys it." Certain depths of torment may be unspeakable. Beyond words, the skeleton on the table communicates violence. Etched in terror, it carries a material message of pain. This is a testimony of bones.

      . . .

AFTER SCILINGO BROKE the silence, Argentine journalist and ESMA survivor Miriam Lewin began investigating death flights. She discovered that the Argentine Coast Guard had purchased five Irish-built planes known as Skyvans. Two were shot down by the British in the Malvinas (Falkland Islands) War. The others had been stored in a hangar at Jorge Newbery airport in Buenos Aires until 1995, when they were sold to private buyers. In 2009, Lewin tracked a Skyvan PA-51 to Fort Lauderdale, where it was being used to shuttle goods between Florida and The Bahamas. She contacted the new owner, who provided her with the complete flight logs, miraculously intact. Poring over the paperwork from 1977, Lewin found records of the death flights, including the pilots' names.

It was, as Lewin said, "a golden discovery," the closest anyone had come to revealing the military's secrets and exposing those responsible. The log from the Skyvan in Florida recorded a flight on December 14, 1977. The plane had taken off from Jorge Newbery airport. Its destination was declared as the naval base of Punta Indio, south of Buenos Aires, where the wide Río de la Plata estuary meets the South Atlantic. The plane never arrived at the base; it returned to Newbery three hours and ten minutes later. The log noted: "Night navigation." The flight is believed to have carried Esther Ballestrino de Careaga, Sister Alice Domon, Azucena Villaflor, and others of the "twelve of Santa Cruz" to their deaths.

Miriam Lewin's investigation was used as evidence in the trial of pilots Mario Daniel Arrú and Alejandro Domingo D'Agostino, who had worked for Aerolineas Argentinas, the national airline, in the years after the dictatorship. In November 2017, both pilots were sentenced to life in prison. It was the first judgment against participants in death flights made in Argentina.

Adolfo Scilingo traveled to Spain, where he gave testimony about the atrocities of the Argentine dictatorship. After describing his role in the death flights, he was arrested on charges of crimes against humanity—for which Spain recognizes no national borders. Although he tried to withdraw his confession, he was indicted by Spanish judge Baltasar Garzón and eventually sentenced to a 1,084-year prison sentence. The amnesty laws in Argentina, which protected Scilingo at the time of his confession, were repealed in 2005, ending impunity and beginning a new era of human rights trials.

In 2010 an Argentine court found former dictator Jorge Rafael Videla guilty of kidnapping, torture, and murder. He was later convicted of the systematic abduction of babies born in clandestine detention centers. Videla died in prison in 2013 while serving a life sentence for crimes against humanity. Among the most important legal proceedings, for its scale and symbolism, was the ESMA "mega case" held from 2012 to 2017. The largest trial in Argentine history, it investigated human rights crimes committed at the clandestine detention center against more than eight hundred victims. Hundreds of witnesses gave testimony about death flights, stolen babies, and the complicity of the Catholic Church. Alfredo Astiz—the Blond Angel of Death—was given a life sentence for crimes against humanity, as were the pilots of the death flights. Since the repeal of the amnesty laws, more than eight hundred people have been convicted of dictatorship-era crimes.

. . .

IT IS GETTING late. We return the shattered bones to their labeled bags and tuck them into the box to be stored among the rest. No name is written on the cardboard, only a code, but Emilia says he has been matched through the DNA database. As soon as the judge signs off, which is just a formality, the family will bury him.

"Que lastima," says Emilia, "What a pity." Then she makes a correction. This is a good thing. This is what everyone works so hard to accomplish, that the bodies be returned to families.

We gather our coats and climb down the stairs. Everyone else has left. On the busy corner, we say goodbye. Walking home alone, I press through the crowds of Once. It is strange to be back in the world of the living after spending the day in the lab. I'm still thinking about the man's body on the exam table, about the slip of the tongue, "que lastima." I know how dedicated Emilia and Adriana are to their work and to the mission to restore the missing to their families. Yet the "que lastima" was honest, too. Any body can be buried. Cemeteries are full of bones. It is a shame to lose these articulate bones and their vivid testimony.

Once his body is buried, his bones will be gone. They will no longer tell their forensic story. All stories require a listener, and this one can only be transmitted body to body, by holding a cranium to better see or running fingers across a fracture to feel. Hand to bone, we (we, the living) understand in a way that words cannot capture what the term "death flight" means.

Later this man's story will be told with words like *They threw him from an airplane*. His shattered bones will become biography, and their fractures will disappear into language. It is a necessary translation. But it is also inadequate. More will be gained, there's no question. So many delicate things had to align to reach the point of his burial. Searching, finding, cleaning, articulating, sampling. Or, from another perspective, the Madres had to gather in Plaza de Mayo on Thursday afternoons. Clyde Snow had to show up in Argentina in his fedora. A group of anthropology students had to be brave or reckless enough to start digging for the disappeared. You could also say that genetic technologies had to be pioneered, DNA databases established, protracted legal battles against impunity fought. And don't forget about the other labors, the work of grief, the years of waiting. For this man to be found, named, and buried has required an epic journey. It seems like a miracle when you think about it.

The crowds of Once have thinned out, on the quieter streets near home, and my mind wanders to *The Iliad* and *The Odyssey*. Some scholars say that the first telling of the Trojan War was in song, performed over days by poet-musicians called aoidoi. Only later did Homer compose the epics, formalizing Odysseus's journey. The story moved from song to story to text. It changed form. It became lighter and more mobile. It traveled farther and faster, circulating around the world. On paper, it sailed through time to the pages about war and its aftermath that I stay up late reading. No one now knows the melodies of the sieges and ships; no one has heard the bards by the night fires sparking toward black skies. In changing form, the music was lost.

The man in the lab's story is changing form, too. After years of being lost, he has been found. He has regained his name. Soon he will be buried with tears and ceremony by those who love and mourn him. Like Odysseus, he will return to those who have waited. As it should be.

But on the quiet street, in the fading light, there is a passing moment of forensic melancholy for the bones that will no longer speak.

CHAPTER 13

The Guarumo Tree

A S I WORKED in the depths of Pozo de Vargas, I wondered why so many mass graves were in wells. In Guatemala, the girl and her dog had been found in a well. In Spain, the bodies of people executed in the civil war were discovered in wells. Remains were disinterred from wells after the 1991–95 war in Croatia. Forensic teams in Cyprus have excavated so many wells that they have developed new technical methods for excavation.

Then it occurred to me that the answer was simple: Wells are holes no one needs to dig; they are graves waiting to be filled. As one academic article puts it, wells are an "easy and obvious choice" for hiding bodies because of their "convenience of use for disposal and perceived inaccessibility for discovery," making them a common site for clandestine burial.

Perhaps the most infamous case of bodies found in a well is the Dos Erres massacre.

In July 1994, the Argentine forensic team arrived at an overgrown patch of land in the northern province of Petén, Guatemala. A village had been burned to the ground twelve years earlier, and all its landmarks had vanished into the undergrowth, but it didn't take long to find the well. A guarumo tree marked the spot, growing from the center of a deep depression in the earth. Tall and straight, its thin trunk expanded into a broad canopy of fat-fingered leaves, the distinctive shape which gives it the name "trumpet tree" in English. This had once been Dos Erres, a thriving hamlet of sixty families.

Invited by Guatemalan human rights groups and families of the disappeared, Patricia "Pato" Bernardi, Silvana Turner, and Darío Olmo of the EAAF cleared the vegetation around the guarumo tree to reveal a circle seven feet in diameter—the opening of the well. Human rights activist Aura Elena Farfán watched alertly while local officials stood nearby. She had begun investigating rumors of a massacre after receiving information that human bones were surfacing from the earth where the town of Dos Erres had once stood.

The team began to dig. After several hours, they'd excavated a hole more than six feet deep but discovered nothing. The public prosecutor left, scoffing that they would never find anything more than dog bones.

. . .

AT 2:30 A.M. on December 6, 1982, a group of Kaibiles, the Guatemalan Army's elite special forces, arrived at Dos Erres. Twenty men disguised as guerrillas entered the sleeping town while the military sealed the perimeter. The community had been accused of collaborating with the guerrillas and hiding twenty-one rifles stolen from the army. Their actual transgression was refusing to participate in Patrullas de Autodefensa (PAC). Called Civil Defense Patrols in English, these local armed groups were organized at the village level as civilian offshoots of the military. They were ostensibly a voluntary force, but participation was coerced under the threat of retaliatory violence. Civil Defense Patrols were directly responsible for atrocities, often in neighboring towns—a deliberate military tactic to turn communities against one another, a strategy that left deep and enduring wounds in rural society. When the commander of the local military base demanded that the men of Dos Erres join a PAC and patrol a nearby village, they resisted. The military interpreted their reluctance to participate in Civil Defense Patrols as a sign of "subversive" sympathies and collaboration with guerrillas.

The soldiers pulled families from their homes, hauling the men to the school and the women to the church. Over the next two days, they massacred more than two hundred people.

The day before the attack, U.S. President Ronald Reagan met with General Efraín Ríos Montt in Honduras, only about three hundred miles from Dos Erres as the crow flies. Reagan called Ríos Montt "a man of great personal integrity and commitment" who was working to "restore democracy" in Guatemala. He promised that the United States would "do all it can to support his progressive efforts."

. . .

AT A DEPTH of about thirteen feet, just after noon, the EAAF unearthed a boy's shirt and a child's rib cage.

. . .

DOS ERRES WAS a new settlement, part of a government program that granted poor families land to grow crops like corn, beans, and pineapples. The town, called "the two Rs" for the last names of the cousins who had founded it, was only about four years old at the time of the massacre. Those murdered at Dos Erres were migrant workers who had come to Petén from other parts of Guatemala looking for a better life. The town had no electricity and no plumbing. Until they dug a well by hand, residents walked six miles with plastic containers to get water from the nearest town.

Kaibil commando Gilberto Jordán initiated the massacre by throwing a crying baby into the well. The truth commission report describes the events that followed: "All of the minors were executed with blows from a sledgehammer to the head, while the smallest ones were held by their feet and smashed against walls or trees." Meanwhile, the Kaibiles interrogated the adults. When the residents denied having any information about the stolen guns—the weapons were never found—the soldiers executed them with gunshots to the head or by smashing their skulls with a sledgehammer. Everyone was thrown into the well. The only known survivors were two boys, aged three and five, kidnapped by the Kaibiles. When no more bodies would fit, the soldiers covered the well with dirt. Some people were still alive and they could be heard screaming and crying from the ground. The following day, soldiers returned to the well. The truth commission report describes that "they found a hand sticking out as if perhaps someone was still alive and was trying to get out." So they added more dirt.

. . .

AT TWENTY-SIX FEET, the forensic team found ten "probable male" skeletons with gunshot trauma. The bodies were fully dressed, and objects retrieved from their pockets—coins from 1977 and 1978, a 1982 calendar, and two identity cards—confirmed that the grave could not date from before 1982. The team was sure there were many more remains at greater depths, but the excavation conditions were perilous. The plans they had made with an engineer in Guatemala City before the project started didn't work out in the field. The backhoe they had rented to remove soil was delayed, and when it finally reached the site, it broke down within hours. The team used a system of ropes tied to trees to lower themselves into the well. Then the rainy season began, and the waterlogged earth walls needed constant reinforcement to prevent them from caving in. A major collapse threatened to bury the team. After twenty days at the site, they halted the excavation.

. . .

EXCAVATING WELLS POSES dangers and technical challenges. "Recovery of victims' remains deposited in wells was the most difficult type of recovery encountered by the identification team," reported experienced forensic archaeologists and anthropologists working in Croatia. The work is treacherous because "all well excavations have a potential to collapse," a risk that grows the deeper the excavation. Teams are counseled to work only "under the supervision of emergency rescue authorities" and to excavate "as quickly and efficiently as possible due to safety risks." Fredy Peccerelli tells me bluntly that inexperienced attempts at excavating wells can be fatal. Discussing an early case that the newly formed Guatemalan team decided not to attempt, he says he's glad they didn't try: "We probably would have died."

At Pozo de Vargas, Santiago and the rest of the team have had to come up with novel methodologies and approaches to excavate the increasing depths of the industrial well. To work safely, forensic teams often collaborate with engineers. Teams have developed a range of technical methods such as "terracing," "ramping," and "pocketing," in which heavy machinery removes the earth around the well to allow for "controlled recovery" of bodies. But in some circumstances, there is no choice other than to lower team members directly into the depths. This last-resort option requires "physical and mental strength."

. . .

THE ARGENTINE TEAM returned to Dos Erres the following May. It was a complex exhumation. Working deep in the well, they discovered that the roots of the guarumo tree had woven themselves through the bones, making it difficult to extract them.

Tiny biting flies called jejenes infiltrated the grave and ate away at skeletons. The site was full of children's bones that were fragile, "like eggshells," said Bernardi.

The forensic team, family members, and human rights groups were harassed and threatened during the exhumation. Equipment was stolen from the excavation site; an army battalion blasted loud military music while they worked; machine guns were fired nearby; the house they were staying in was pelted with stones. They received death threats. The prosecutor in charge of the case asked to be removed because he was worried about his family's safety.

When the exhumation reached forty feet, they had recovered the remains of 162 people, including 67 children younger than twelve. The remains showed evidence of violence, including skull fractures and bullet holes. Some bones bore "fractures compatible with lesions caused by firearm projectiles" in the cranium and thorax. Ballistic evidence associated with the remains included spent cartridges from Galil rifles, a weapon commonly used by the army. In several cases, plastic cords were found knotted around the bones of hands and feet, and ropes were tied around the cervical vertebrae of the neck. There were also peri- and postmortem fractures consistent with damage from dumping the bodies in the well, the pressure of the other bodies, and the weight of the earth fill used to cover the site. The excavation revealed that women and children had been killed first and men last.

At the very bottom of the well were the small bones of a newborn.

Witnessing the exhumation, Aura Elena often had to run into the woods to cry, shattered by what she saw. "The massacre of Dos Erres marked me for my entire life," she said years afterward. "It marked me because they first began their massacre by killing the children."

• • •

BY THE TIME Aura Elena began investigating Dos Erres, she was already a well-known human rights advocate. Her brother, Rubén Amílcar Farfán, a student at the University of San Carlos active in the Guatemalan labor party, disappeared in 1984. Searching for Rubén at the city morgue and La Verbena Cemetery, Aura Elena saw hundreds of mutilated bodies, revealing the scale of the state terror. Decades later, Rubén's photo and documents pertaining to his disappearance were discovered among the moldering papers of the National Police archive. His name appeared on a list with the number 300 printed beside it—a code for execution. His remains have not been found.

In the immediate aftermath of Rubén's disappearance, Aura Elena united with other family members of the missing to establish two of the most influential human rights associations in Guatemala: the Mutual Support Group (GAM) and the Association of Families of the Detained and Disappeared (FAMDEGUA). These organizations, along with the National Coordination of Widows of Guatemala (CONAVIGUA), saw exhumation as essential in their fight for justice and accountability. In a joint statement, they said, "Peace will not come to Guatemala as long as the remains of our massacred relatives continue to be buried in clandestine cemeteries. . . . For this reason, we continue to demand the formation of forensic teams." Clyde Snow began investigating mass graves in Guatemala in the 1990s, supporting the efforts of families and human rights organizations. The Guatemalan team was established in 1992. Forensic experts from Argentina, Chile, and the United States supported the new team's work and training.

There were a staggering number of graves to exhume. The nascent Guatemalan team made an agreement with the Argentine team to collaborate. While the EAAF worked in Dos Erres, the Guatemalan team was exhuming other sites, including a mass grave in the village of Plan de Sánchez, where Clyde Snow helped search for more than 250 people, primarily women, children, and the elderly, massacred in 1982.

. . .

CLYDE SNOW MENTORED the Guatemalan team just as he had the Argentine team, returning to the country many times. Snow told anthropologist Victoria Sanford, who had joined the Plan de Sánchez exhumation in late July 1994 (where she was learning not to faint or vomit), that she was lucky to be working with the Guatemalan team, who were the best possible teachers. Snow told her, "The thing that most people don't understand is that these guys are the real experts. We may have more advanced technology in our labs in the United States, but these guys have more experience with the bones than anyone else. Look at all the graves here. The bones don't lie and these guys know what they say. They are the real professionals of forensic anthropology."

For all his forensic experience, Snow was shocked by what he saw. "If anyone wanted to commit murder and get away with it, they should come to Guatemala."

. . .

FREDY PECCERELLI LEFT Guatemala when he was nine years old. His father, a competitive bodybuilder and international judge in the sport, had received death threats, so in 1980, the family moved to New York. "At the time, I thought it was the worst thing that ever happened to me," he tells me. His neighborhood in the South Bronx was tough, but a world away from the political violence the family had fled. Growing up near Yankee Stadium, Fredy had a pretty typical American childhood, punctuated by the wins and losses of his favorite team, shielded from the genocide unfolding in Guatemala.

It wasn't until he was a student at Brooklyn College and read the book *I, Rigoberta Menchú* for a class that he started to think deeply about the country his family had fled. Rigoberta Menchú had recently won the Nobel Peace Prize, and her testimonio recounted how La Violencia impacted her K'iche' Maya community and formed her as a human rights activist. Even after Fredy set down the book, her story stayed with him, particularly her descriptions of the Maya Cosmovision. Testimonio had begun its work on him, with its way of changing those who hear it as certainly and as profoundly as chopping wood and carrying water shape bone. He decided he needed to go to Guatemala. He was already an anthropology major, so he resolved to find a way to spend the summer in the jungles of Petén searching for lost archaeological treasures, like an Indiana Jones from the South Bronx. Fredy organized a trip with his college anthropology club to attend the annual meeting of the American Anthropological Association. At the convention center in Atlanta, he sought out famous Mesoamerican archaeologists, but he found their talks less thrilling than he had imagined. Looking around for an interesting panel, he wandered into a session on "exhuming the past" and sat in the front row. The speaker, dressed in a blazer, cowboy boots, and a fedora, sauntered to the lectern. Clyde Snow snapped to the first slide of his talk: a photo of the Argentine forensic team excavating an N.N. grave. "I was struck by lightning right there," says Fredy.

After the talk, Fredy asked how he could get involved. Clyde said he would be teaching a class in Guatemala in January; maybe his colleagues there would agree to let Fredy come along. Two months later, Fredy was standing in a mass grave with Clyde Snow and the Guatemalan forensic team.

He never left. He eventually became the director of the team. Fredy learned, in material detail, in earth and bone, about the violence of Guatemala he'd been shielded from growing up. As

he made sense of his parallel lives between the Bronx and El Quiché, he developed the habit of calculating which Yankees game
he'd been watching when a particular massacre occurred. As if to
decipher how the same hours could hold both, how life is simul-
taneous and incommensurate.

Fredy was mesmerized by the way Clyde Snow did the work.
No gloves or Tyvek suits, no police tape, no distance between the
team and the family. He talked to everyone, explained everything about the process to the families, smoked like a chimney,
and stayed up late drinking single malt scotch with the team. He
didn't care much about publishing papers—he cared about finding the dead. He was warm and down-to-earth and cared deeply
about the families, but he also knew how to keep a professional
distance. He taught Fredy to "work in the day and cry at night,"
just like he had instructed the students in Argentina.

Clyde Snow had first come to Guatemala at the behest of families of the disappeared to investigate specific cases, including
the murder of Myrna Mack. But he kept coming back, just like he
had in Argentina. Clyde trained Latin American forensic teams,
but the teams taught him, too. Fredy tells me that Clyde always
said, "You guys are the experts. I'm here to help you and to learn
from you." At the time, this pronouncement astonished Fredy. "I
was like—learn from us?" What could a new team teach an expert forensic scientist? But Clyde was always learning. At the
first exhumations in Argentina, he had been taken aback to see
families at the gravesites and in the lab. By the time he arrived in
Guatemala, he was a strong advocate for community-centered
forensic practice.

. . .

AFTER SEVERAL YEARS of exhuming graves in rural areas of
Guatemala, where the brunt of the violence was carried out in
massacres like the one at Dos Erres, Clyde asked Fredy, "What

about the disappeared?" What about the people who had vanished without a trace? Investigating a massacre poses many challenges, but it is a "closed context" case, like an airplane crash. At least in rough terms, the team knew who they were looking for: the sixty families who lived in Dos Erres; the 250 women, children, and elderly people from Plan de Sánchez. In Guatemala, there were so many massacres that the team didn't need to search for bodies to exhume. For the most part, communities had an idea where the mass graves were, even if they kept it to themselves for fear of reprisal.

But Clyde had a point: In urban areas, like Guatemala City, there weren't massacres; there were disappearances. Activists, students, union leaders, journalists—people like Rubén Amílcar Farfán—had vanished, abducted from homes, schools, and city streets. No one knew where these bodies were.

Clyde said, "Maybe it happened like in Argentina."

Fredy asked, "How did it happen in Argentina?"

Clyde explained the junta's tactic of secretly burying the disappeared in N.N. graves, nameless plots in urban cemeteries.

. . .

FREDY AND CLYDE, dressed in his cowboy boots and hat, arrived at the office of La Verbena Cemetery and asked to see their records. "Of course, Dr. Snow," said the administrator. "There's just one problem, we only have registers from 1977 to 1986," naming the span of years at the height of state violence.

"That's just fine," said Clyde.

Sure enough, poring over the ledgers, Clyde found increased death rates corresponding to periods of increased political violence. Working in Argentina, he had pioneered methods of forensic statistics to calculate excess deaths, which had revealed a steep spike in N.N. graves during the dictatorship. In the cemetery logbooks in Guatemala, Clyde discovered statistical evidence. He also found descriptive entries about gunshot wounds, signs of ligature strangulation, and marks from edged instruments. The registries described bodies burned beyond recognition and corpses with their hands lopped off, presumably to prevent identification.

"We've just solved a thousand murders," Clyde told Fredy. But when they went to La Verbena to search for unnamed burial plots, known as X.X. graves in Guatemala, the gravediggers said the bodies weren't there anymore; they had been dug up long ago to make space. The workers showed Fredy and Clyde where the remains had been transferred, pulling open the covers of the ossuaries. Clyde took one look at the thousands of bones in their depths and said it was impossible. "Just tell the families that they're here." The same situation had arisen on occasion in Argentina. These cases were considered lost causes. A forensic report explained, "Regrettably, some of the remains have already been exhumed from their individual tombs by cemetery personnel and sent to the general ossuary of the cemetery." It went on to say, "When placed in the ossuary, we can no longer recover the remains, since they are mixed with thousands of other bones."

But, at La Verbena, Fredy decided to try. "I sometimes have difficulty separating between laser-focused and obsessed," he tells me. Clyde calculated there to be 889 victims of state terror among what they estimated to be 16,000 remains in ossuaries. "I was called crazy many times," Fredy says. "It borders on impossible."

On the first day of the La Verbena exhumation, the team invited families of the missing, who made a circle around one of the bone wells. People made speeches and threw flowers into the ossuary. Then something unscripted happened. The families began to shout the names of the dead. They began to scream and cry the names of those they had lost. It went on for almost an hour.

Fredy was shaken by the outpouring of grief, fury, and hope. He knew one thing: The exhumation might be impossible, but it had to be done.

The technical challenges were enormous, and the team had to engineer new approaches. On one of Clyde's visits, he and Fredy suited up in full hazmat gear and belayed into the depths of one of the ossuaries. Dangling over the tangle of remains, Clyde surveyed the scene. Then he reached down. He plucked a skull from the mass of bones, holding it up to show Fredy the bullet hole. Among the tens of thousands of remains, he had found a murder victim on his first try. "That was Clyde. He was bigger than life," says Fredy.

. . .

THE DOS ERRES trial began on July 25, 2011. Silvana Turner from the Argentine team testified that 171 human remains had been recovered from the well and surrounding areas. Forty percent of the bodies recovered were children aged zero to twelve. Members of the Guatemalan team presented genetic evidence identifying the two young boys abducted by the Kaibiles as Ramiro Osorio Cristales and Oscar Alfredo Ramírez Castañeda, the sole survivors of the massacre. The Guatemalan team also presented findings from a field analysis of Dos Erres made in 2010, when they discovered, among the bones, a sledgehammer.

Three Kaibiles and the commander of the local military base were found guilty for their roles in the massacre of Dos Erres. Each man was sentenced to 6,060 years in prison.

. . .

AFTER THE MASSACRE and before the military burned Dos Erres to the ground, a handful of neighbors visited the destroyed settlement looking for friends and family. It was a few days after the attack. They found stray dogs, scattered belongings, and a man hanging from a tree, his face covered with flies. María Esperanza Arreaga ventured to her brother's house, which had been ransacked. She looked under the bed and found her nieces' shoes stuffed with socks, and she burst into tears. Saúl Arévalo searched for his father. He found his work boots lying on the ground. Then he noticed that an abandoned well on his family's property had been covered with dirt. It looked recent. He saw bloody clothing strewn nearby. He cut a branch from a guarumo tree to probe the well. The branch sank deep into the soft, fresh soil. He understood where his father and everyone else in Dos Erres had vanished to. He fell to his knees and wept.

The branch Saúl left in the well took root and flagged the site for the Argentine forensic team when they came to exhume the mass grave twelve years later. Known for its fast growth, the guarumo is valued for its straight, hollow trunk, which can be used to make weapons like blowguns, and for the medicinal properties of its leaves, used to treat maladies like heart problems. Like the tree that marked it, the exhumation of Dos Erres possessed force and healing through the stories it brought to light and the evidence it brought to trial.

But there are no simple remedies in Guatemala. Five days after the Dos Erres sentencing, Fredy received a note scrawled in red ink, threatening him and other team members for their part in the convictions. It read: "Anthropology Foundation sons of bitches . . . When you least expect it you will die. Revolutionaries your DNA will be of no use."

. . .

THE END OF La Violencia did not bring an end to violence. Human rights leader Rosalina Tuyuc says, "The end of the armed conflict was really just a ceasefire, there was no de-structuring of the political, economic, and military system, which today remains intact." The largest massacre since the end of the armed conflict occurred as the Dos Erres trial was about to begin in May 2011, just a few miles from where the town once stood. Members of the Zetas entered Los Cocos ranch at night, looking for its owner, who allegedly owed the cartel a debt. They bound and interrogated the farmworkers. When the workers denied having any information about the owner's whereabouts—he was never found—the Zetas gruesomely tortured and executed them. Neighbors arriving the following day to buy milk and cream found twenty-seven bodies, most decapitated, strewn around the ranch. The workers murdered at Los Cocos had no involvement in narcotrafficking; they were migrants who had come to Petén from other parts of Guatemala looking for a better life, just like the inhabitants of Dos Erres decades before.

Among the Zetas who directed and carried out the Los Cocos massacre were ex-Kaibiles. The 1996 peace process did not dismantle the Kaibiles. In the years after the Dos Erres massacre, Kaibiles were named to top military and political positions, including the presidency, under Otto Pérez Molina, a former soldier in the special forces. Kaibiles also formed close ties with narcotrafficking groups, training them in their brutal methods. Petén, where Dos Erres and Los Cocos are located, is also home to Kaibil bases. It is a busy corridor for trafficking. Groups like the Zetas—and the ex-Kaibiles working with them—smuggle drugs and prey on migrants making their way to Mexico's "La Bestia"—the infamous train running north to the U.S. border. As sociologist Gladys Tzul Tzul notes, whether Guatemalans stay in their country or try to go north, they are vulnerable to armed groups who "commit crimes and acts of terror against citizens and against those trying to flee such terror."

As the massacre at Los Cocos hit news headlines, the parallels with Dos Erres were widely noted. Tzul Tzul observed that Los Cocos was part of a larger pattern: "The violence of today can be interpreted as a continuation of the genocidal war" of La Violencia. Claudia Paz y Paz, Guatemala's attorney general at the time of the Dos Erres trial, said of the Los Cocos massacre, "We can't separate what is happening now from what happened during the war and how structures were created at that time to generate terror."

Officials investigating the massacre at Los Cocos showed journalist Óscar Martínez a photo of the crime scene. Studying the image of the mutilated dead splayed across the field, Martínez was struck by "the bodies still wearing their heavy work boots," much as I had been affected by the boots in the mass grave at Xolosinay. The Kaibiles blur into the Zetas; poor people continue to move north to Petén and beyond; La Violencia changes form, but the structures of terror endure.

CHAPTER 14

The Well

I'M WORKING WITH SANTIAGO in the depths of Pozo de Vargas. Shifting into a new position, I lose my balance and slip. I step on a rib. It audibly cracks under my weight. I look at Santiago in panic. I've left my foot where it landed in a misguided attempt to do no more damage, as if it were a stab wound and I am not removing the knife. "It's okay," he says, offering me a hand. I retreat to the small patch of packed earth between bones, the lily pad where I'd been balancing.

"Don't worry," he says, seeing I'm upset. "It doesn't matter." I know this is true in a certain sense. The bone has remained in place. When the fracture is analyzed in the lab, it will be apparent that it is postmortem damage. But the sensation of the bone cracking leaves me disturbed. It reverberates through me, ringing in my body like a bell, part sound, part sensation, part visceral horror—shaking me awake to the reality that I am at the bottom of a dark well filled with the dead, the violently killed.

I'd like to run away, but there's no easy way to leave the Pozo. With the sound of the bone still vibrating through me, I get back to work. Better not to think about leaving. In Guatemala, I used to worry about fainting, vomiting, and crying. Those worries have been replaced by a more subtle, hard-to-pin-down unease that buzzes in the background, like the sensation of cracking bone trailing through my body.

I catch myself wondering what happens if you are working in the well when the electricity goes out. Power cuts aren't unusual in Argentina. The industrial lights would go dark. The air pump would stop. The elevator would not work. We would have to use the ladder. I could climb out, I tell myself. I wonder how often wells collapse. It's been standing since the nineteenth century, I tell myself.

As I clean mud from a cranium, his perfect beautiful teeth smiling from the dirt, a spider appears and crawls across the mandible into the cavity of the skull. I am as freaked out as if I'd just seen it slip between Santiago's lips. A skeleton has no inside or outside. A spider cannot threaten a mandible, only a mouth. This boy in the mud is beyond danger. But my heart races.

Extracting a graceful radius, I suddenly wonder what happened to these bodies when they decomposed. Where has all the muscle and skin and blood gone? The dirt in the Pozo is packed tight around the bones. In archaeological terms, it is a "muddy matrix" composed of soil and organic matter. Dense and moist, it reminds me of flesh. Bodies are organic matter. Is this flesh-mud?

I begin to avoid the Pozo. On the way to Tucumán, my bus breaks down an hour outside of Buenos Aires. The trip is canceled. They send us back to Retiro station in an out-of-commission city bus with no shock absorbers that smells like engine oil. Bouncing back to the city with my backpack on my knees, I'm relieved, happy not to go, even if it is only a temporary reprieve.

One Sunday afternoon, alone in the little apartment I've rented in Tucumán, I'm standing at the kitchen counter, reading a book and eating a sandwich. Suddenly, I can't swallow. My throat is closed, as if I've been painlessly stung by a bee in the esophagus. I try to drink water, and it spews from my mouth onto my shirt. I tell myself to stay calm, that my airway is clear, as I position my ribs against the back of a chair to give myself the Heimlich maneuver. Suddenly it passes. I search "inability to swallow" online, and I see that, among cancers and goiters, it is associated with panic attacks.

I wouldn't describe what I feel as *panic*, but there is a constant undercurrent of dread. I realize that I no longer dream about bones. I'm not sure when I stopped. I no longer dream at all. I get headaches. I break out in a rash on my neck that climbs across my face before spreading to the folds of my arms and the backs of my legs. In quick succession, my neck cramps, my shoulder freezes, and my elbow swells up like a large, bruised mango. When I dig, my wrist aches. I think of how in Guatemala, Alvaro told me that many team members develop chronic skin conditions. But I don't think this is happening because of fungal spores or injury. It is my body in revolt.

In anthropology, much has been written on "somatization," physical expressions of psychological suffering, "idioms of distress" in which bodily afflictions are forms of communication. I know that symptoms can be narratives and codes, with context and subtext. I know that illness can weave together the biological and social. That the body has its metaphors and insistence on meaning. It makes sense to me that there is a message written in these pains and rashes, but I don't know what it says. Or maybe I just don't want to read it. Instead, I push on. When I eat, I take small bites, chewing deliberately so I don't choke. When I work, I dig with my good hand, avoiding my painful wrist.

. . .

DESCENDING INTO THE Pozo in the yellow elevator, I sometimes think we are entering the land of the dead. It is not a place of torment, not a Christian hell, though the human evil that created this place evokes that, too. It is a more ancient underworld, like Hades. In the utter darkness held at fragile bay by the lights, in the thin air and muffled sounds, it belongs to another dimension. It is the world of the dead, quite literally. Some say that at the spot where Hades kidnapped Persephone into the underworld, a well appeared. Like that mythical world with its contracts written in pomegranate seeds, the Pozo has its own rules and laws. Here, time is reversed; we move toward the past, digging through the years, the strata of violence. Sometimes time stands still. I think of folktales where a man is captured by the fairies. In their underground world, he feels that only a few hours have gone by, but when he returns to his village, he finds his parents dead and his sisters old and withered. We might take the elevator out of the Pozo and discover that a hundred years have passed. We would surface and crumble to dust.

. . .

WHY ARE THESE vital young people buried here? I am thinking of the bones, of the disappeared, murdered in the prime of their lives. But I am also thinking of the team. Santiago, El Oso, and the others who work in the depths, day in and day out. They've been excavating for more than a decade. They have spent years of their lives laboring underground. The hours of a lifetime pile up in the Pozo. In photos from the first days of the excavation, they look round-faced and younger. They age and change. Theirs is human time, but the bones belong to geological time. I think of something Mimi Doretti said to *The New York Times* in 1987, when she was in her midtwenties and the EAAF was only a few years into its work. She said the exhumations were important, but they would not do it forever: "We all have other ambitions, ideas more connected to life." Thirty-five years later, Mimi is investigating disappearances in Mexico.

. . .

ONCE, AT DINNER with friends and colleagues from the Argentine and Guatemalan teams, Clyde Snow had too much to drink and got a little weepy. It was unlike him, a man who knew how to handle his liquor and deflect too much navel-gazing with quips and wit. But that night, he turned to Fredy with tears in his eyes and said, "I'm sorry." He apologized for getting him started in forensics. Otherwise, Fredy would have been mayor of New York by now. He told Mimi that she would have been Argentina's most famous writer. He went around the table, apologizing and imagining alternative lives. Everyone was laughing, and Clyde was crying. The expression "poner el cuerpo" is hard to translate into English. Literally, it means "to put the body," and it has the sense of "give it your all" and "put yourself on the line." It is total commitment, often to a political cause, sometimes to the point of self-sacrifice. In the search for the dead and disappeared, finding bodies requires teams to poner el cuerpo. Bodies for bodies.

· · ·

CROUCHED IN FRONT of the dead in the Pozo, there is only one task: clean the dirt off the bones, centimeter by centimeter. It must be done. The dead cannot stay here. It has its own powerful logic, like myth. Like Psyche sorting a mountain of millet and poppy seeds. Like two sisters gathering the scattered pieces of Osiris's body. Like making a rope of ashes.

· · ·

MAYBE THE POZO itself brings on these strange thoughts. I am not dreaming of the dead, but the Pozo conjures fever-dream moments: time running toward the past, feeling buried alive, the bloody, muddy matrix. In many sacred traditions, wells carry a magical charge. They are places of Christian pilgrimage, as they were for the ancient Celts. Throwing offerings of coins, beads, pebbles, and buttons into the depths of "wishing wells" for healing and good luck is an ancient and widespread practice. It was described by Pliny the Younger. Even now, we continue the custom when tourists throw thousands of dollars' worth of coins into the fountains of Rome every day. I grew up believing that you could see stars in daylight from the bottom of a deep well. This is a very old idea, and apocryphal. Aristotle believed it. So did my dad. In European folklore, the faces of the dead appear in the still water of wells, as do the faces of the future beloved. Wells, like caves, are linked to fertility rites. The well can be the tunnel of death and the channel of birth.

Wells are entrances to other worlds. In ancient Greece, the underground belonged to deities. Mystery initiations and prophecies were accompanied by the descent into caves and underground chambers. Sages and seers descended seeking "ecstatic illumination." Some scholars argue that underground spaces bring on altered states of consciousness. Studies show that even brief periods of sensory deprivation can invoke trancelike states.

If a well can be a kind of temple, exhumation can be a kind of meditation. Many sacred traditions have practices of contemplation on death and the bodies of the dead. In Thailand, monks meditate on decaying corpses, as the Buddha himself was said to have done, sitting in a grave among bones. Contemplating the dead, the meditators say of their own bodies: "This body, too. Such is its nature, such is its future, such its unavoidable fate." The Islamic philosopher and mystic al-Ghazali encouraged picturing the decay of a loved one's body: "Now the worm has devoured his tongue, how he used to laugh, while now the dust has consumed his teeth." In Catholicism, pilgrims visit the dead bodies of saints, and holy relics of tooth and bone. In the small graveyard near my father's house in New England, where I used to like to take walks, you can read a headstone that says: "As you are now, so once was I. As I am now, soon you shall be. Prepare yourself to follow me." In art, paintings of skulls and bones are "memento mori," which means "remember that you have to die." Even philosophy is a meditation on death; according to Cicero: "To philosophize is to learn how to die." My field too may have this calling: "Can an anthropology of dying teach a conscious-ness, yours or mine, how to dissolve into emptiness, and thus how to live?" asks anthropologist Robert Desjarlais.

We are not kneeling in Pozo de Vargas to meditate. Still, spending hours in the small space, unable to move freely, with no distraction, slowly working to free the bones of a slain genera-tion from the earth, cannot help but be a contemplation of death and violence.

• • •

WHEN WE WORK together in the damp hush of the well, in the spotlight of the LED, Santiago tells me about following Inca roads through the salt-white deserts of the north to look for cave paint-ings and burial mounds. On the surface, he loads satellite images on his phone and points out the ancient tracks carved in the land-scape. Aboveground, Santiago is commanding. He moves boul-ders, shovels drainage trenches, delivers documents to the courts, interviews with journalists, drafts grant applications, and talks to families. Santiago gets things done. But in the well, he is reflec-tive, as if we've descended to somewhere closer to the springs of memory. In fragments and snapshots, he tells me about his child-hood, his difficult father, and his early love of archaeology. He tells me about the Reiki and healing workshops he takes on the weekends, about the Inca roads and where they lead him. From his stories, I can't help but feel that working in the Pozo has changed him from the angry young man he once was to who he is now—patient, beneficent, wise, the spiritual center of the team.

• • •

I TRAVEL TO Bogotá, Colombia, to attend a Red Cross conference on the "legal, technical, and psychosocial aspects of enforced dis-appearance." Delegates from forensic teams, government agen-cies, human rights groups, and organizations of families of the missing pack the basement meeting rooms of a downtown hotel. In keynote talks, speakers flash PowerPoint graphs quantifying horror and calculating death. There are presentations from across Latin America; there are mass graves everywhere. On a break, as we balance our cups and saucers and read one another's name tags, someone makes a gallows-humor joke: "It's a good field to get into," he says. "There's always work."

I attend a workshop with psychologists and social workers from Guatemala. The presenters know Zulma, who taught me so much about testimonios and "taking the lid off sadness" when we worked together in El Quiché. I have begun to understand that the Guatemalan and Argentine approach that centers families and works closely with communities is much admired but still a work in progress in other countries, which rely on more top-down approaches.

In the middle of a talk on forensic pathology, I get a message from Santiago: "We found something." On a break, I hurry up the stairs to the hotel lobby, where there is better reception. Santiago tells me that this morning, just a few hours ago, they found a piece of paper in the Pozo. It was in the pocket of a young man. In the years of work, in the depths excavated, in the tens of thousands of fragments of bone found—there has never been paper. How can something so fragile have survived? "It's a miracle," he says. He is emotional: elated, tearful. He tells me they've stopped work to decipher it. They can make out some of the words. They think it is a song.

I have missed the miracle. I go back to the basement. The next talk has already started; a mass grave marked in quadrants is projected on the wall.

· · ·

IN THE EARLIEST days of my fieldwork, I watched the washing of bones. The forensic practitioner's touch was gentle and precise. I thought of a photo I'd seen of a widow in Greece washing the bones of her husband. His body had been disinterred in a ritual to read the state of his soul from the state of his bones. Then his bones were washed in wine, wrapped in cloth, and placed in a wooden box in an ossuary. In the lab, bones were washed in water, wrapped in paper, and placed in a cardboard box in storage. My mind staggered for a moment, caught: Which was the act of faith?

This question can be asked of the cardboard boxes of bones kept in storage. The dirt of the grave brushed from the bones and saved for the families. The careful sorting of the bones of sixteen thousand people in the ossuaries of La Verbena Cemetery. The 130 feet excavated at Pozo de Vargas. The 93,030 reference samples analyzed in the Western Balkans and the 1,800,000 tons of debris workers sorted through after 9/11 to collect fragments of tooth and bone as small as peas.

One of the hallmarks of lamentation is its excess. Talking becomes screaming, singing becomes wailing. Mourners act out their pain on their own bodies, tearing their clothes and hair, beating their chests, even inflicting injuries. This intensity sets it apart from other forms of public witnessing. Lamentation is communication as it reels toward the unsayable, the inexpressible pain of loss. I see in practices of exhumation, in the lengths gone to recover the dead after annihilating violence, something of this excess. The enormous forensic undertakings are scientific and legal efforts, but they are also expressions of pain and acts of faith. As a postcard pinned to an office door at the FAFG forensic laboratory says: "Archeology is my religion."

· · ·

IN COLOMBIA, AT a visit to a suspected mass grave in a city garbage dump, a forensic team member tells a story about the first time mothers of the disappeared came to the site. They had waited a long time to be allowed access because of local politics and ostensible concerns over safety. When they were finally admitted, several mothers sat on the ground and covered themselves in dirt. The forensic team members who witnessed this act were puzzled and even disturbed, but one mother told them, "The ground where my son lies is sacred ground."

. . .

EXHUMATION BEGINS BY marking off space. The area is closed to the public and may be roped off with bright plastic tape. It is marked, measured, and mapped. Tarps, blackboards chalked with dates and codes, grids of string, cards with arrows pointing north, and red flags spring up at the site. Archaeologists survey the area, using everything from probing sticks to ground-penetrating radar. Data is recorded with laptops, paper forms, cameras, and GPS. What had hours before been a nondescript space—an empty lot, an abandoned school, a military base, an industrial well, an ossuary, a parking garage, its history of terror remembered or forgotten—is transformed into an exhumation site.

This transformation has practical and symbolic effects. Practically, it allows remains to be efficiently recovered and systematically documented, maintaining legal chains of custody for evidence. Symbolically, it marks the area as a space of death. Exhumations are inseparable from catastrophic violence, from a society torn apart. The "very act of cordoning off and securing an area of violence and horror," writes archaeologist Zoë Crossland, and "bringing scientific techniques and practices to bear on a locus of disorder and destruction has a powerful symbolic force." At the heart of exhumation's power is its promise to restore order through science. The yellow tape is a flag against impunity and forgetting. The presence of a forensic team claims that chaotic and violent events of the past, once hidden, can be witnessed and brought back into official memory.

With backhoes, shovels, pickaxes, and buckets, teams search the ground and bring the dead back into the fold of the living. Just as we don't bury the dead for purely scientific and legal reasons—to avoid the spread of disease or because it is required by law to do so—we don't unbury the dead for purely rational and functional reasons either. We exhume bodies for the same reason we bury bodies—because they are our dead.

Burial is not the only way to care for the dead, of course, and cremation or any other funeral ritual can be substituted here. But I refer to burial because it is ancient and symbolically potent. Death and burial are closely linked in English and the Romance languages. The word "posthumous," defined as "after death," means "after earth"—after burial. Linguistically and symbolically, death and burial are joined. Some scholars even trace a connection between the word "human" and the Latin terms for earth and burial: "humus" and "humando." As scholar Robert Pogue Harrison says, "To be human is to bury." To be human is also to exhume.

• • •

INVESTIGATING GENOCIDE IN Kibuye, Rwanda, in 1996, forensic anthropologist Clea Koff worked under difficult conditions. Crouched in a mass grave, light-headed from the heat and stench, she exposed a body: "She was lying on her left side, her back to the wall of the grave, and the radiating fractures from a hole on the left side of her head reached around her cranium like fault lines." Finding pink necklaces wrapped around the cervical vertebrae, "I forgot my discomfort. . . . Now I was totally focused. This woman had been alive once, not so long ago, and had fastened the necklaces herself." A journalist pulled Koff away from the work and asked what she'd been thinking about in the mass grave. Flashing on the woman with the pink necklaces, Koff answered that she'd been thinking, "We're coming. We're coming to take you out."

At an excavation in Campo Pineda, Honduras, a settlement inhabited more than a thousand years ago, archaeologist Rosemary Joyce worked in a trench that had been looted for its ancient treasures. She writes, "As I troweled down the narrow wall, clumps of dirt pulled away from something off-white. I carefully picked at the object with finer tools and soon realized I was looking at a row of teeth in the side of a jaw, part of a body so small that it was obviously a juvenile, curled up as if sleeping. How could I leave this child there, to weather out of the pit wall or, worse, to be torn out carelessly and tossed aside by people searching for the rare carved marble vases that were the biggest payoff for local subsistence diggers? I could not." Joyce worked for hours in the heat, staying behind as the rest of the team left, "tracing the pit that contained this small body, talking to it as I did so."

In these cases, the dead make demands on the living, appealing through the visceral register, below the surface of conscious thought. Working through heat and exhaustion, these anthropologists feel compelled to move bodies from intolerable burial sites. The dead beseech care, they lloran y gritan, they cry and scream. They are offered words of comfort. They are told: "We're coming," which is what we say to someone in distress: We're on our way, almost there; hold on. The gut feelings that the dead elicit in the living about where their bones belong and where they cannot stay offer clues about the deeper meaning of exhumations.

• • •

IN MOST CULTURES, funeral rituals require the presence of a body. Exhumations are necessary precursors to funerals because they return remains to families and communities. Archaeologist Zoë Crossland observes that because exhumations make funerals possible, they are therefore "part of the production of the sacred."

I would go further. I have come to see exhumations as sacred practices of caring for the dead. In other words, exhumations don't just allow funeral rituals; they *are* funeral rituals.

. . .

PERHAPS THE MOST influential text on death and ritual was written by a young French student named Robert Hertz, a protégé of Emile Durkheim and Marcel Mauss, founding thinkers of anthropology and sociology. Hertz's 1907 essay, eventually published in a book called *Death and the Right Hand,* argues that death is a dangerous, disordering event for societies, and that funeral rituals restore order.

Hertz sees funerals as rites of passage, a transition in which the dead move from their place among the living to a new status as an ancestor. "Death is not completed in one instantaneous act," Hertz writes. Death is a process. The efforts of the mourners, as they perform funeral rituals, allow the dead to complete their journey. Violent and untimely deaths, which Hertz calls "bad deaths," are especially difficult because the "transitional period is indefinitely prolonged, and death is without end," leaving mourners in pain and the dead unsettled. "Bad deaths" require special funeral rituals.

Robert Hertz died in battle in World War I at the age of thirty-four. Emile Durkheim and Marcel Mauss wrote obituaries for him, but I have found no record of the funeral rituals performed for the "bad death" of a young man killed violently.

Hertz believed that death involves three actors: the soul, the corpse, and the mourners. Exhumations add a new actor, the scientist, to this trinity. Death demands burial, and "bad deaths," like disappearances and massacres, demand exhumation.

To say that exhumations are connected to rituals and rites of passage may seem disconcerting. To claim that forensic science is a means to attentively care for our ancestors may seem baffling. Rituals and ancestors are most often assigned to the realm of the irrational and non-modern. They fit into categories of the "other"—other times and other places. Yet, if you take a closer look at modern relationships between the living and the dead, "rituals" and "ancestors" are terms that fit quite well.

For a start, consider beliefs about "dignity" and "respect" for human remains. Anthropologist Talal Asad observes that corpses are legally required to be treated with dignity, an obligation with ties to "ancient beliefs about life after death" that grant the dead body "quasi-'religious' status" and "a measure of sanctity." This status is made explicit in a report outlining "best practices" for forensic exhumation: "Respect the remains; they are part of the deceased person and as such are in some way sacred."

Widespread interest in genealogy, evident in the popularity of DNA ancestry test kits and TV series about celebrities tracing their family roots, also reveals something about the modern relationship between the living and the dead. Documenting family history through archival research and genetic testing is "a form of tribute by ordinary living people to their ancestors," in the words of anthropologist Fenella Cannell. When we map our family tree, part of what we are doing is honoring the dead. The most obvious aspect of genealogy is also its most neglected: Ancestry is about ancestors.

Like genealogy and laws about the dignified treatment of the dead, exhumation is connected to rituals and ancestors. It offers a scientifically sophisticated and technologically advanced means of caring for the dead. This is not to say that exhumations are *only* rituals or *only* about ancestors. Exhumations are also scientific practices with crucial legal and political implications for human rights. But these aspects are widely recognized, whereas their ritual aspects are not. We must look beyond law and science to examine exhumation as "more than a technical process," as anthropologist Katherine Verdery urges; to consider the "meanings, feelings, the sacred, ideas of morality, the nonrational" that are always part of our dealings with the dead.

To neglect a full recognition of the sacred and ritual aspects of exhumations is to suffer an emaciated understanding of what makes them significant and their crucial role in societies fractured by violence. Typically, the success of an exhumation is assessed by technical and legal metrics: how many bodies are recovered and identified, and what role forensic evidence plays in prosecuting human rights abuses. These are crucial outcomes. But they do not capture the full contribution of exhumations.

The very act of marking off an excavation site bears witness to past violence. Even when bodies are never found, the act of looking for them is meaningful. Even when remains cannot be identified, a code on a cardboard box holds the memory of a name and the possibility of restoring it. Even when exhumations "fail"—as measured by narrow scientific and legal metrics—they matter. Their power is in the searching, not just the finding.

. . .

IN THEIR BLOODY wake, the dictatorships of Argentina and Guatemala left a task at once impossible and urgent: finding the disappeared. The dictators burned the logs that recorded the names of their victims and shredded the maps that marked their graves. They hid their archives and kept their silence.

Yet forensic teams started looking for the missing. They came armed with teaspoons and plastic buckets. Courageous, they showed up. They started in their youth and have spent their lives searching.

. . .

SANTIAGO PRESSES THE button and the yellow elevator descends. At excavation level, there are no bones, just dirt, rocks, and chunks of mortared brick. Among the debris, we find a few fragments of bone, sifted down from other layers: a chubby toe bone, a piece of cranium stained orange by the decomposing iron of the railyard trash dumped in the well. El Oso explains that this could be the end of the bodies, but more likely, it is a "tapa"—a layer of fill dumped to hide the grave and dull the smell. It isn't the first tapa they've encountered. Removing the fill is backbreaking work. Boulders and large sections of mortared bricks have to be broken apart with a sledgehammer before they can be lifted out. Day after day, the team hauls out rocks and bricks. Rocks and bricks.

. . .

IT IS NEARLY time to leave Argentina. I dread going back to the manicured lawns and temperature-controlled archives of the university, where everything I've learned and experienced in Argentina and Guatemala will be reduced to scholarly articles, pinned like butterflies. The roiling of real life will be transformed into an academic still life, what the French call "nature morte": dead nature. The sacred will be razored away from the science. The profile will be separated from the vase. There will be no room for ghosts and dreams. The violence written on bones will be abstracted, terror theorized, grief footnoted. All perfectly correct, and painfully incomplete. The research questions will be answered in academic arguments.

The real questions, the ones that brought me here, aren't reducible to claims.

What is to be learned from the catastrophe of history? Can inheritances of violence be transformed? Where are the wellsprings of courage found? How do we go on in the face of incalculable loss?

These are the questions the dead ask us. They cannot be answered or ignored. We can only live into the questions. For this, we have science and law. For this we have ritual, dreams, and each other. W. H. Auden wrote: "Through art, we are able to break bread with the dead, and without communion with the dead, a fully human life is impossible." The living need what the ancestors ask us and ask of us. There aren't answers, but there are lessons.

In the Pozo and in the lab, the dead whisper to me that it didn't have to be this way. The massacres, secret prisons, and hidden graves, all the terror and loss. Another world is possible. On a burning planet, pockmarked by mass graves, it is hard to have much faith. But my work among the dead has taught me that even in the face of violence and terror and breakdown, even at the bottom of the well, there is something—a movement of life, an impulse for justice, a kind of pulsating love. It can be blocked and slowed, and often is, but it will never be eradicated or killed because it flows through everything: ecstatic, electric, unstoppable. It moves in us, through us, and between us, as we surface between ancestor and progeny, between those who came before and those who will come after, as we float together in this vanishing moment—in the fragile possibility of remaking the world.

. . .

AFTER WEEKS OF pulling rocks and bricks out of the depths of Pozo de Vargas, the team finds bodies again. The exhumation continues. In the timeless time, in the constant earth-temperature, in the moldering smell, in the hush and crinkle of the hazmat suits, the team puzzles bones from the muddy matrix. Centimeter by centimeter, with brushes and trowels, they work against impunity and forgetting. They remove the dead from where they must not be. It continues, this forensic care of the ancestors, this labor of justice for the future. As I write this, Santiago, El Oso, and the rest of the team are still exhuming the Pozo. The work is not finished.

• • •

ON A CLOUDY afternoon, I took the yellow elevator up for the last time and stepped into the sweet air.

CLYDE SNOW DIED IN 2014. He was honored by the Argentine forensic team, the Guatemalan forensic team, and teams worldwide. An obituary in *The Washington Post* compared him to Sherlock Holmes and called him "the country's best-known grave-digging detective." Before his death, Clyde asked Fredy to place some of his ashes in the earth of Guatemala with the victims of La Violencia.

Fundación de Antropología Forense de Guatemala (FAFG) completed the "impossible" exhumations of the bone wells at La Verbena Cemetery. The team continues to search for those killed in disappearances and massacres during La Violencia. They also increasingly work internationally. The team shares their vision of family-centered forensic practice and helps build local capacity in countries including Mexico, Colombia, Sri Lanka, and Bangladesh (with the Rohingya refugee population), inspired by the memory of Clyde Snow's commitment to empowering community-led human rights work.

Equipo Argentino de Antropología Forense (EAAF) continues forensic investigations in Argentina and around the world. In 2020, the team was nominated for a Nobel Peace Prize for their trailblazing work searching for the disappeared. In 2021, they joined with the Abuelas de Plaza de Mayo and Argentina's National Commission for the Right to Identity to launch an international campaign to identify children of the disappeared who were abducted during the dictatorship, and who may be living in

Europe, North America, and other places outside of Argentina. The team is now headquartered in the Memory and Human Rights Space, formerly ESMA. The infamous clandestine detention center has been converted into a community center and exhibition space, housing a museum, the National Archive of Memory, and offices for human rights groups.

El Colectivo de Arqueología, Memoria e Identidad de Tucumán (CAMIT) is still exhuming bodies from Pozo de Vargas, among the largest known mass graves in Latin America. They have overcome significant technical challenges from flooding and faced budgetary cuts that left the team unpaid for many months. They are determined to excavate the well until all remains have been recovered. In 2019, the team published a book about their work, *Arqueología Forense y Procesos de Memorias: Saberes y Reflexiones Desde las Prácticas.*

After my fieldwork, I knew I would never be able to "work in the day and cry at night." My research now focuses not on excavating mass graves but on trying to prevent them. The Guatemalan police archive and the connection it revealed between surveillance, disappearance, and genocide left a deep impression on me. I began investigating the human rights implications of emerging technological forms of mass surveillance, like facial recognition technology. Archives of surveillance are increasingly spectral and more dangerous for their invisibility. "Fichas," the cards that marked someone as suspicious, are now virtual, automated, and algorithmic. The Madres of today—journalists, activists, and others organizing for human rights in oppressive political conditions—are not betrayed by a kiss but by their phones and scans of their faces.

ACKNOWLEDGMENTS

I OFFER MY DEEPEST GRATITUDE to the families who shared their experiences with such generosity, patience, and courage. Your testimonios and stories changed me, stay with me, and contain more than one book, or a library of books, could ever hold.

To the forensic team members who so warmly welcomed me to accompany them, thank you for all you have taught me—from details of taphonomy to the meaning of solidarity.

My heartfelt thanks go to Fredy Peccerelli, executive director of Fundación de Antropología Forense de Guatemala (FAFG). From the first days of field school to the last pages of this book and far beyond, your work teaches me what justice in action looks like. I've been searching for the right word to describe your dedication and I don't think one exists that captures your unflagging commitment to the families of the missing, and to the dignity of the dead. Thank you for sharing your expertise and experiences with such honesty and warmth. Erica Henderson has been a tireless champion and trusted guide. Thank you for imparting your expert knowledge and, most important, your wisdom with such kindness.

I am grateful to Dr. Luis Fondebrider, founding member of Equipo Argentino de Antropología Forense (EAAF) and president at the time of my research, now leading the forensic unit of the International Committee of the Red Cross in Geneva, Switzerland. There could be no interlocutor more magnanimous and perceptive, who brings such political nuance, historical context, and philosophical and literary depth to every conversation. Thank you for sharing your extraordinary expertise, insights, and boundless sense of compassion.

At CAMIT, Víctor Ataliva and Ruy Zurita's dedication to archaeology in service of human rights is exceeded only by their warmth and goodwill. Your profound commitment to families, your tenacious pursuit of truth, your grace under pressure, and your tireless work to forge connections between science and justice are an object lesson in how to remake the world. Special thanks to Ruy for the steady flow of patient explanations and reading suggestions he has offered during the course of writing this book.

I extend my gratitude to Rosalina Tuyuc and Feliciana Macario of Coordinadora Nacional de Viudas de Guatemala (CONAVIGUA), Susana Navarro García of Equipo de Estudios Comunitarios y Acción Psicosocial (ECAP), Mario Polanco of Grupo de Apoyo Mutuo (GAM), Alberto Fuentes Rosales of Archivo Histórico de la Policía Nacional (AHPN), Nicolas Pedregal of Equipo Argentino de Trabajo e Investigación Psicosocial, and members of Asociación Civil Abuelas de Plaza de Mayo, Asociación Madres de Plaza de Mayo, Madres de Plaza de Mayo Línea Fundadora, Familiares de Desaparecidos y Detenidos por Razones Políticas, and Hijos e Hijas por la Identidad y la Justicia contra el Olvido y el Silencio (HIJOS), for enriching my understanding of your crucial work. My deep thanks to Ana María Careaga and Father Carlos Saracini for the privilege of ongoing conversations. My gratitude to Josefina Molina for sharing her important and perceptive insights.

At Stanford, Tanya Luhrmann shared her expansive view of the potentials of anthropology and the possibilities of writing.

Thank you, Tanya, for your scholarship and encouragement; you saw this book before I did, and your belief in me brought it forth.

Lochlann Jain cultivates an approach to intellectual inquiry at once urgent and playful, serious and sly, rigorous and daring. Thank you, Lochlann, for your open invitation to experiment in a living laboratory of analysis and empathy, and for your staunch and nimble support.

I thank Robert Pogue Harrison for arriving with conversations that ricochet between the subterranean and the celestial, when such a gift was most needed, and for his abiding graciousness.

Courses and conversations with Angela Garcia, Ximena Briceño, Duana Fulwiley, Liisa Malkki, Paulla Ebron, Sharika Thiranagama, and Thomas Blom Hansen shaped my thinking in important ways. I thank Ellen Christensen and Shelly Coughlan for their invaluable support.

At Berkeley, I am grateful for the mentorship of Charles Briggs and for courses and conversations with Nancy Scheper-Hughes, Sabrina Agarwal, Laurie Wilkie, Thomas Laqueur, and Stefania Pandolfo. I also thank Ned Garrett for being a perpetual oasis.

I give special thanks to my doctoral cohort: Misha Bykowski, Jennifer Hsieh, Saree Kayne, Vivian Chenxue Lu, Johanna Markkula, Kathryn Takabvirwa. I am also grateful for time spent turning over ideas with: Jess Auerbach, Rachel Carmen Ceasar, Rachel Cypher, Nisrin Elamin, Leslie Grothaus, Shakthi Nataraj, Emily Ng, Dilshanie Perera, Raphaëlle Rabanes, Nethra Samarawickrema, Grace Zhou, and many other thoughtful and artful anthropologists remaking the field from inside and outside. The anthropology community, and far beyond, has been deeply touched by the immeasurable loss of colleagues Martin Fortier, who was illuminated by an unforgettable sense of intellectual discovery, and Sam Dubal, whose commitment to research rooted in justice remains a beacon.

I am indebted to the brilliant and convivial SSRC DPDF cohort "Critical Approaches to Human Rights": Samar Al-Bulushi, Jian-Ming Chris Chang, Evelyn Galindo, Christoph Hanssmann, Grégoire Hervouet-Zeiber, Austin Kocher, Laura Matson, Jaime Morse, Justin Perez, A. Marie Ranjbar, and J Sebastian, mentored by Amy Ross and Chandra Lekha Sriram, who is deeply missed.

My editor, Aubrey Martinson, is gifted in the art of balancing vision and practicality, finding maps in the stars and landmarks on a map. I can't think of a more invaluable set of skills for bringing a book into the world. Thank you, Aubrey, for your sense of direction and sense of adventure. I'm deeply grateful for such a wonderful traveling companion. This book exists because of you.

My agent, Lucy Cleland, has nurtured this work with exquisite care and enormous skill. From the beginning, she grasped the spirit and shape of this work with a clarity that bordered on augury. Her pivotal interventions are as concise, forceful, and meaningful as hinges on a door; they open the way. Immeasurable thanks, Lucy, for your fierce intelligence, your resolute belief in the importance of telling these stories, and your trusted counsel.

I extend my profound gratitude to John Lee, whose generous spirit, faith in my work, and sensitive reading have nourished this project from the first to the last. Thank you, John, for everything.

Stacy Patwardhan provided discerning notes and unwavering encouragement. Sheryl Fragin gave fruitful comments and an all-important first push. Rob Latham at LARB, Greg Downey at *Ethos*, and Ariel Evan Mayse of Stanford gave important feedback on earlier versions and other forms of this work.

I could not have navigated the long road from idea to proposal to fieldwork to book without the generosity of many people who offered reading suggestions, musing on methodology, introductions to colleagues, and much more. I extend special thanks to: Diego Jemio, Florencia Aranda, Marcelo Medina, Eric Jimenez López, Davette Gadison, Cristian Silva Zuniga, María Celeste Perosino, María Epele, Anita Jemio, Raquel De Maestri, Vinciane Despret, Adam Rosenblatt, Zoë Crossland, Robin Reineke, Alejandra Gomez Cano, Marta Fernandez, and Marten Boekelo. Thank you to fact-checker extraordinaire Andy Young, "one of the four kindest people in the world," for your keen eyes and quick wit. I'm grateful to Elizabeth Oglesby for her generosity in helping me better understand the life and work of Myrna Mack Chang. I was rereading Diane Nelson's powerful, magical book *Reckoning: The Ends of War in Guatemala* when I learned of her death. I will never forget how, when I reached out to her for advice during fieldwork, she responded with such wisdom and luminous empathy. We will continue to be transformed by her work.

In research, writing, and life, I'm grateful for steadfast friends and colleagues: Tori Kjer, Kiran Nimmagadda, Victoria Walker, Véronique Guillemot, Rand Abu Ghanimeh, Meredith Root-Bernstein, Siri Lamoureaux, Louise Hickman, Igor Rubinov, Alexandra Albert, Richard McKay, Stephanie Hare, Anjali Mazumder, Natalie Jones, Robert Desjarlais, Aidan Seale-Feldman, Luis Felipe Murillo, Aurélie Lafond, Ivan Piotrowski, and Emily-Jane Dawson. Thank you, David Mimoun, for starwatching; Margaux Fitoussi, for figs and wasps; and Livia Garofalo, for poetry and possibility. I am grateful to Joaquin Bulacio for the leap of faith.

Everything goes to my family, far and wide, with special gratitude to my mother, Karen Kirchberg, and my stepfather, Michael Kirchberg, for the many hours of conversations, many pages of reading, and many miles you've traveled. Your love is a blessing. I am lucky to spend my life among the Kirchberg and

Hagerty crews. I wish my father were here to read this. His big heart lives on in Mary, Megan, Clyde, and Ezra and their families. I also wish the wise and beloved Barry Krasner were here to read this. May his memory be a revolution.

I owe many other thanks, too, for the web of kinship and friendship that sustains me.

The research that this book is based on was supported by fellowships and grants from the Mellon Foundation, the Wenner-Gren Foundation, the Social Science Research Council, and the National Science Foundation.

vii **"We have always said":** Rosalina Tuyuc, quoted in Fredy Pecce-relli and Erica Henderson, "Forensics and Maya Ceremonies: The Long Journey for Truth in Guatemala," in *The Routledge Handbook of Religion, Mass Atrocity, and Genocide,* eds. Sara E. Brown and Stephen D. Smith (Routledge, 2021), 318.

Introduction: Articulating Bones

xiii **"There are 206 bones":** Martin Weil, "Clyde Snow, Forensic An-thropologist Who Identified Crime Victims, Dies at 86," *The Washington Post,* May 16, 2014.

xv **The linguistic root:** References to etymology in this section are drawn from the Oxford English Dictionary, *OED Online* (Oxford University Press, March 2022).

xv **governments in Latin America:** Works that discuss state terror-ism and genocide in Latin America and its aftermath from com-parative and/or multicountry perspectives include Juan E. Corradi, Patricia Weiss Fagen, and Manuel Antonio Garretón, *Fear at the Edge: State Terror and Resistance in Latin America* (University of California, 1992); Marcia Esparza, Daniel Feierstein, and Henry R. Huttenbach, eds., *State Violence and Genocide in South America: The Cold War Years* (Routledge, 2009); Krujit Koonings, *Societies of Fear: The Legacy of Civil War, Violence and Terror in Latin America* (Zed Books, 1999). For a comparative discussion of state terror beyond Latin America, see Jeffrey A. Sluka, ed., *Death Squad: The Anthropology of State Terror* (University of Pennsylva-nia Press, 2010).

xvi **Latin American forensic teams have led the field:** Silvia Dutrénit-Bielous, *Forensic Anthropology Teams in Latin America* (Routledge, 2019); Luis Fondebrider, "Forensic Anthropology and the Investigation of Political Violence," in *Necropolitics: Mass*

Graves and Exhumations in the Age of Human Rights, eds. Francisco Ferrándiz and Antonius C.G.M. Robben (University of Pennsylvania Press, 2015).

Chapter 1: A Lovely Grave for Learning

3 **La Violencia:** I use the term "La Violencia" following my interlocutors, the Guatemalan Commission for Historical Clarification (CEH), and the work of anthropologists and historians including Victoria Sanford, Linda Green, Virginia Garrard-Burnett, and Daniel Rothenberg. However, it is a contested term, in part because it may act to render the perpetrators as invisible forces and those killed as nameless, passive victims, making violence seem like something that "just happens," like weather. As truth commission reports *Memory of Silence* (CEH) and *Guatemala: Never Again* (REMHI) make clear, and as discussed in this book, the Guatemalan state carried out genocidal violence against its citizens, particularly Maya communities. For a thoughtful discussion of these themes, see Elizabeth Oglesby, "Educating Citizens in Postwar Guatemala: Historical Memory, Genocide, and the Culture of Peace," *Radical History Review* no. 97 (2007).

3 **"Don't faint. Don't vomit":** Victoria Sanford, *Buried Secrets: Truth and Human Rights in Guatemala* (Palgrave Macmillan, 2003), 31.

3 **cycles of life associated with decay:** James T. Pokines, Ericka N. L'Abbe, and Steven A. Symes, eds., *Manual of Forensic Taphonomy* (CRC Press, 2021).

4 **lines from *The Tempest*:** William Shakespeare, *The New Oxford Shakespeare: The Complete Works* (Oxford University Press, 2016).

5 **five hundred years of colonial conquest:** Greg Grandin, "Five Hundred Years," in *War by Other Means: Aftermath in Post-Genocide Guatemala*, eds. Carlota McAllister and Diane M. Nelson (Duke University Press, 2013); W. George Lovell, "Surviving Conquest: The Maya of Guatemala in Historical Perspective," *Latin American Research Review* 23, no. 2 (1988); Victor Perera, *Unfinished Conquest: The Guatemalan Tragedy* (University of California Press, 1995); W. George Lovell, *A Beauty That Hurts: Life and Death in Guatemala* (University of Texas Press, 2010).

5 **"force of great suffering":** Munro S. Edmonson, *Heaven Born Merida and Its Destiny: The Book of Chilam Balam of Chumayel*

(University of Texas Press, 2010), 110. For a Guatemalan account, see Matthew Restall and Florine Gabriëlle Laurence Asselbergs, *Invading Guatemala: Spanish, Nahua, and Maya Accounts of the Conquest Wars* (Penn State University Press, 2007).

5   **"misery and affliction":** Edmonson, *Heaven Born*, 110.

7   **Commission for Historical Clarification:** Comisión para el Esclarecimiento Histórico (CEH), *Memoria del Silencio* (CEH, 1999). An abridged version was published in English as *Memory of Silence: The Guatemalan Truth Commission Report*, ed. Daniel Rothenberg (Palgrave Macmillan, 2012).

7   **200,000 dead:** CEH, *Memory of Silence*, 179.

7   **45,000 people had been disappeared:** Amnesty International, "City of the Disappeared—Three Decades of Searching for Guatemala's Missing," November 19, 2012.

7   **More than a million people suffered forced displacement:** Inter-American Commission on Human Rights, "Fifth Report on the Situation of Human Rights in Guatemala," April 6, 2001.

7   **626 massacres:** CEH, *Memory of Silence*, 45.

7   **430 villages razed:** Larry Rohter, "Guatemalan Indians Return from Exile, Warily," *The New York Times*, January 15, 1996.

7   **93 percent of the documented abuses:** CEH, *Memory of Silence*, 179.

7   **More than 80 percent of the victims:** Ibid. The exact number is 83.3 percent.

7   **chronicled by human rights groups:** Human rights reports include Amnesty International, *Guatemala: Massive Extrajudicial Executions in Rural Areas Under the Government of General Efraín Ríos Montt*, July 1982; Americas Watch Committee and Physicians for Human Rights, "Guatemala: Getting Away with Murder" (Human Rights Watch Publications, 1991).

7   **"Even if 30 forensic teams worked":** Fernando Moscoso, interviewed at the Plan de Sánchez exhumation site in 1994, quoted in Grahame Russell, Sarah Kee, and Ann Butwell, *Unearthing the Truth: Exhuming a Decade of Terror in Guatemala* (EPICA/CHRLA, 1996).

8   **formal systems of training and accreditation:** In Latin America, the first professional certification exams took place in 2012 under the auspices of the Asociación Latinoamericana de Antropología Forense and the Directorio Latinoamericano de Antropología Forense. Nicholas V. Passalacqua and Marin Pilloud, "The Need to

Professionalize Forensic Anthropology," *European Journal of Anatomy* 25 (2021).

9 **most violent cities:** James Painter, "Crime Dominates Guatemala Campaign," BBC News, May 10, 2007; International Crisis Group, "Guatemala: Squeezed Between Crime and Impunity," *Latin America Reports,* June 22, 2010; Tiziano Breda, "Curtain Falls on Guatemala's International Commission Against Impunity," International Crisis Group, September 3, 2019.

9 **violence rapidly escalated:** United Nations Office of Drugs and Crime (UNODC), International Homicide Statistics Database, "Intentional Homicide (per 100,000)—Guatemala," 2006–2010.

9 **murders left unsolved:** David Grann, "A Murder Foretold," *The New Yorker,* March 28, 2011; Leonardo Goi, "Nearly All Crimes in Guatemala Go Unpunished: CICIG," *InSight Crime,* April 6, 2017.

9 **"a good place to commit a murder":** Philip Alston, "A Good Place to Commit Murder," in *The Guatemala Reader: History, Culture, Politics,* eds. Greg Grandin, Deborah T. Levenson, and Elizabeth Oglesby (Duke University Press, 2011).

9 *New Yorker* **article on crime:** Grann, "Murder Foretold."

9 **what "postwar" really meant:** Philip Alston, "Report of the Special Rapporteur on Extrajudicial, Summary or Arbitrary Executions," United Nations Human Rights Council, April 16, 2008; Carlota McAllister and Diane M. Nelson, *War by Other Means: Aftermath in Post-Genocide Guatemala* (Duke University Press, 2013); Kevin Lewis O'Neill and Kedron Thomas, *Securing the City* (Duke University Press, 2011); Victoria Sanford, "From Genocide to Feminicide: Impunity and Human Rights in Twenty-First Century Guatemala," *Journal of Human Rights* 7, no. 2 (2008).

9 **many of the same actors:** Grann, "Murder Foretold"; Steven Dudley, "Élites y Crimen Organizado en Guatemala: la CICIG," *InSight Crime,* March 28, 2017; International Commission Against Impunity in Guatemala (CICIG), *Sixth Report of Activities of the International Commission Against Impunity in Guatemala,* 2013.

9 **"sells an illusion":** Associated Press, "Guatemalan Capital's Wealthy Offered Haven in Gated City," *The Guardian,* January 9, 2013.

10 **Guatemala City morgue:** Consulate General of the United States in Guatemala, "Disposition of Remains," *Factsheet,* 2016.

10 **no more room in the municipal cemeteries:** Kevin Lewis O'Neill,

"There Is No More Room: Cemeteries, Personhood, and Bare Death," *Ethnography* 13, no. 4 (2012).

12 **California grows more than half:** California Department of Food and Agriculture, "An Era of Productivity and Perseverance," *CDFA Report,* 2019–2020.

12 **88 percent of the state's farmworkers:** "California Findings from the National Agricultural Workers Survey (NAWS) 2015–2019: A Demographic and Employment Profile of California Farmworkers" (NAWS, January 2022).

13 **"Guatemalans had been migrating":** James Verini, "How U.S. Policy Turned the Sonoran Desert into a Graveyard for Migrants." *The New York Times Magazine,* August 18, 2020.

13 **Crossing the border can be deadly:** See Francisco Cantú, *The Line Becomes a River: Dispatches from the Border* (Riverhead Books, 2018); Jason De León, *The Land of Open Graves* (University of California Press, 2015); Óscar Martínez, *The Beast: Riding the Rails and Dodging Narcos on the Migrant Trail* (Verso Books, 2014).

13 **U.S. government secured:** Wayne A. Cornelius, "Death at the Border: Efficacy and Unintended Consequences of US Immigration Control Policy," *Population and Development Review* 27, no. 4 (2001); Timothy J. Dunn, *Blockading the Border and Human Rights: The El Paso Operation That Remade Immigration Enforcement* (University of Texas Press, 2010); Joseph Nevins, *Operation Gatekeeper and Beyond: The War on 'Illegals' and the Remaking of the U.S.–Mexico Boundary* (Routledge, 2010); Verini, "How U.S. Policy Turned the Sonoran Desert into a Graveyard for Migrants."

13 **"a killing machine":** De León, *Land of Open Graves,* 3.

13 **"mass disaster" at the border:** Alberto Giordano and M. Katherine Spradley, "Migrant Deaths at the Arizona–Mexico Border: Spatial Trends of a Mass Disaster," *Forensic Science International,* August 12, 2017; Daniel Martinez et al., "A Continued Humanitarian Crisis at the Border: Undocumented Border Crosser Deaths Recorded by the Pima County Office of the Medical Examiner, 1990–2012," Binational Migration Institute, University of Arizona, June 2013.

14 **buried in unmarked graves:** Clyde Collins Snow, Fredy Armando Peccerelli, José Samuel Susanávar, Alan G. Robinson, and Jose

Maria Najera Ochoa, "Hidden in Plain Sight: X.X. Burials and the Desaparecidos in the Department of Guatemala, 1977–1986," in *Statistical Methods for Human Rights* (Springer, 2008).

14 **thrown from planes:** Horacio Verbitsky, *Confessions of an Argentine Dirty Warrior*, trans. Esther Allen (New Press, 2005).

14 **bodies are burned:** "Countless Human Remains Found at Cartel 'Extermination Site' Near U.S. Border as Mexico Can't Account for Nearly 100,000 Missing," CBS News, February 28, 2022; Lizzie Wade, "Were the Bodies of 43 Missing Students Burned at a Dumpsite?," *Science*, March 10, 2016.

14 **3,781 people:** April 2022 figures from the Fundación de Antropología Forense de Guatemala. See also The Forensic Anthropology Foundation of Guatemala, *Annual Report 2020* (FAFG, 2020).

14 **1,400 sets of remains:** Antonella Bernetti, "Cómo Trabaja el Equipo Argentino de Antropología Forense, Rol Clave en la Identificación de Desaparecidos: 'Tenemos un Compromiso Asumido,'" *El Destape*, July 27, 2022; Marc Raboy, "Memory, Truth, and Justice as Argentina Honours the Victims of State Terrorism," Oxford University Press blog, March 24, 2022.

16 **turned into a testimonio:** There is a vast literature on testimonio, including John Beverley, *Testimonio: On the Politics of Truth* (University of Minnesota Press, 2004); Natalia De Marinis and Morna Macleod, "El Testimonio en Latinoamérica: Usos y Destinos," *Desacatos: Revista de Ciencias Sociales* 62 (2020); Margaret Randall, John Beverley, and George Yudice, *The Real Thing: Testimonial Discourse and Latin America* (Duke University Press, 1996).

16 **Using pseudonyms is standard:** The field debates the use of pseudonyms, like many other theories and methods. See Erica Weiss and Carole McGranahan, "Rethinking Pseudonyms in Ethnography: An Introduction," *American Ethnologist*, December 2021. For a discussion of people's mixed feelings about using their real names in testimonios shared with anthropologists, see Victoria Sanford, "Breaking the Reign of Silence: Ethnography of a Clandestine Cemetery," in *Human Rights in the Maya Region: Global Politics, Cultural Contentions, and Moral Engagements*, eds. Pedro Pitarch, Shannon Speed, and Xochitl Leyva So (Duke University Press, 2008).

16 **Exhumations can be political flashpoints:** The account of Ríos

Montt's arrival in Rabinal is from Julie Stewart, "A Measure of Justice: The Rabinal Human Rights Movement in Post-war Guatemala," *Qualitative Sociology* 31, no. 3 (2008).

16 **twenty documented massacres:** CEH, *Memory of Silence*, 71.

Chapter 2: Forensic Lamentations

23 **Recovery of Historical Memory:** Arzobispado de Guatemala, *Guatemala: Nunca Más: Impactos de la Violencia, Informe Proyecto Interdiocesano de Recuperación de la Memoria Historica* (REMHI), Oficina de Derechos Humanos del Arzobispado de Guatemala, 1998. An abridged version was published in English: Archdiocese of Guatemala, *Guatemala: Never Again* (Orbis Books, 1999).

23 **"Families have the right to exhume":** Archdiocese of Guatemala, *Guatemala: Never Again*, 317.

23 **"Learning the truth is painful":** Bishop Juan Gerardi, "Discurso de Monseñor Juan Gerardi con Ocasión de la Presentación del Informe REMHI," transcript of a speech delivered at the Catedral Metropolitana, April 24, 1998.

24 **the military assassinated Bishop Gerardi:** For an absorbing and detailed account of the investigation and the wider political context, see Francisco Goldman, *The Art of Political Murder: Who Killed Bishop Gerardi?* (Atlantic Books, 2010).

24 **"Death to the anthropologists":** Amnesty International, "Guatemala: Further Information on Fear for Safety/Death Threats" (Index Number: AMR 34/009/2006), March 16, 2006. Threats aren't limited to teams. Writing in 1998, anthropologist Judith Zur observed, "Most villagers are too frightened to avail themselves of their legal right to petition for the exhumation of clandestine cemeteries. People whose jobs bring them into contact with petitioners receive death threats," including civilian officials, local judges, and lawyers. Judith N. Zur, *Violent Memories: Mayan War Widows in Guatemala* (Routledge, 2019), 222.

24 **Since its founding in 1992:** The team's original name was Equipo de Antropología Forense de Guatemala, or EAFG. For simplicity, I use their current name, Fundación de Antropología Forense de Guatemala (FAFG), throughout.

24 **the dead need their everyday things:** For more on the armed

conflict and funeral rituals, see Fernando Suazo, *La Cultura Maya y la Muerte: Daño y Duelo en la Comunidad Achi de Rabinal* (ECAP, 2010); Pau Pérez-Sales and Susana Navarro García, *Resistencias Contra el Olvido: Trabajo Psicosocial en Procesos de Exhumaciones* (Editorial Gedisa, 2007).

25 **Bodies were left for days:** Zur, *Violent Memories,* 80.

26 **poorest parts of a poor country:** World Bank, "Guatemala: Poverty and Equity Brief," April 2022.

26 **Maya communities and culture:** As summarized by a truth commission: "The army systematically attacked cultural, spiritual, and religious elements of life that held deep meaning for the people.... And, they desecrated temples, religious imagery, and sacred sites." CEH, *Memory of Silence,* 49.

26 **humans were formed from corn:** Dennis Tedlock, *Popol Vuh: The Definitive Edition of the Mayan Book of the Dawn of Life* (Simon and Schuster, 1996), 163–64; for a translation in verse, see Michael Bazzett, *The Popol Vuh: A New English Version* (Milkweed Editions, 2018).

26 **grains of maize are passed down:** For more on transmitting strategies of maize cultivation, see Avexnim Cojti, Cesar Gomez, and Bia'ni Madsa' Juárez López, "United in Tradition as Peoples of the Corn," *Cultural Survival,* September 2019. For recent research on maize and migration, see Ann Gibbons, "The Maya—and the Maize That Sustained Them—Had Surprising Southern Roots, Ancient DNA Suggests," *Science,* March 22, 2022.

26 **buried with maize in their mouths:** Robert J. Sharer, *The Ancient Maya* (Stanford University Press, 1994), 673; Andrew K. Scherer, *Mortuary Landscapes of the Classic Maya: Rituals of Body and Soul* (University of Texas Press, 2015), 76; Alberto Ruz Lhuillier, *Costumbres Funerarias de Los Antiguos Mayas* (UNAM, Seminario de Cultura Maya, 1968), 162; Suazo, *La Cultura Maya y la Muerte,* 16, 33.

26 **"massive assault":** David J. McCreery, "Coffee and Class: The Structure of Development in Liberal Guatemala," *Hispanic American Historical Review* 56, no. 3 (1976): 457. See also David McCreery, *Rural Guatemala, 1760–1940* (Stanford University Press, 1994).

26 **twentieth century, Maya land:** Alberto Alonso-Fradejas, "Land Control-Grabbing in Guatemala: The Political Economy of Contemporary Agrarian Change," *Canadian Journal of Development*

Studies 33, no. 4 (2012); Giovanni Batz, "Ixil Maya Resistance Against Megaprojects in Cotzal, Guatemala," *Theory & Event* 23, no. 4 (2020); Greg Grandin, *The Last Colonial Massacre: Latin America in the Cold War* (University of Chicago Press, 2011); Emma Pauliina Pietilainen and Gerardo Otero, "Power and Dispossession in the Neoliberal Food Regime: Oil Palm Expansion in Guatemala," *The Journal of Peasant Studies* 46, no. 6 (2019). For a well-written personal account exploring connections between land reform and the armed conflict, see Daniel Wilkinson, *Silence on the Mountain* (Duke University Press, 2004).

26   **continue in the twenty-first century:** Jennifer Devine and Diana Ojeda, "Violence and Dispossession in Tourism Development: A Critical Geographical Approach," *Journal of Sustainable Tourism* 25, no. 5 (2017); Catherine Nolin and Jaqui Stephens, "'We Have to Protect the Investors': 'Development' and Canadian Mining Companies in Guatemala," *Journal of Rural and Community Development* 5, no. 3 (2010); Simona V. Yagenova and Rocío Garcia, "Indigenous People's Struggles Against Transnational Mining Companies in Guatemala: The Sipakapa People vs Goldcorp Mining Company," *Socialism and Democracy* 23, no. 3 (2009); Megan Ybarra, *Green Wars: Conservation and Decolonization in the Maya Forest* (University of California Press, 2018).

27   **"looking under the same earth":** Gladys Tzul Tzul, "Rebuilding Communal Life," *NACLA Report on the Americas* 50, no. 4 (2018): 404.

27   **"the land where the dead rest":** Ibid.

27   **structural violence:** Paul Farmer, "An Anthropology of Structural Violence," *Current Anthropology* 45, no. 3 (2004).

27   **describe it as "hateful":** Quoted in Diane M. Nelson, *Reckoning: The Ends of War in Guatemala* (Duke University Press, 2009), 3.

27   **where you get malaria:** Ibid.

28   **human rights recognized:** UN General Assembly, "Universal Declaration of Human Rights," *UN General Assembly* 302, no. 2 (1948); see also "The Right to Health" (OHRC Factsheet No. 31) and "The Right to Adequate Food" (OHRC Factsheet No. 34).

28   **"What do all of these victims":** Paul Farmer, *Pathologies of Power* (University of California Press, 2004), 255.

28   **"when we talk about":** Irma Alicia Velásquez Nimatuj, "Struggles and Obstacles in Indigenous Women's Fight for Justice in Guatemala," *Portal* 11 (2016): 25; Lieselotte Viaene, "Life Is Priceless:

Mayan Q'eqchi' Voices on the Guatemalan National Reparations Program," *International Journal of Transitional Justice* 4, no. 1 (2010); Denis Martínez and Luisa Gómez, "A Promise to Be Fulfilled: Reparations for Victims of the Armed Conflict in Guatemala," Queen's University Belfast, *Reparations, Responsibility, Victimhood in Transitional Societies*, August 2019.

29 **marks of structural violence:** Jared S. Beatrice, Angela Soler, Robin C. Reineke, and Daniel E. Martínez, "Skeletal Evidence of Structural Violence Among Undocumented Migrants from Mexico and Central America," *American Journal of Physical Anthropology* 176, no. 4 (2021).

30 **religious differences:** Virginia Garrard-Burnett, *Terror in the Land of the Holy Spirit: Guatemala Under General Efraín Ríos Montt 1982–1983* (Oxford University Press, 2010); Nelson, *Reckoning*.

31 **Catholics were singled out:** CEH, *Memory of Silence*, 57, 74; Nelson, *Reckoning*, 180.

31 **Ríos Montt established "model villages":** Asociación para el Avance de las Ciencias Sociales en Guatemala, *Política Institutional Hacia los Desplazados en Guatemala* (AVANSCO, 1990); Mikkel Jordahl, *Counterinsurgency and Development in the Altiplano: The Role of Model Villages and the Poles of Development in the Pacification of Guatemala's Indigenous Highlands* (Guatemala Human Rights Commission, 1987); W. George Lovell, "Surviving Conquest: The Maya of Guatemala in Historical Perspective," *Latin American Research Review* 23, no. 2 (1988); Beatriz Manz, *Paradise in Ashes* (University of California Press, 2004), 155–82.

31 **shared Maya identity:** Demetrio Cojtí Cuxil, "The Pan-Maya Movement," in *The Guatemala Reader: History, Culture, Politics*, eds. Greg Grandin, Deborah T. Levenson, and Elizabeth Oglesby (Duke University Press, 2011); Diane M. Nelson, *A Finger in the Wound: Body Politics in Quincentennial Guatemala* (University of California Press, 1999); Tzul Tzul, "Rebuilding Communal Life"; Kay B. Warren, *Indigenous Movements and Their Critics: Pan-Maya Activism in Guatemala* (Princeton University Press, 1998).

33 **Inhumations require ritual creativity:** For another account of ritual creativity at a community inhumation, see Clara Duterme,

"Honouring, Commemorating, Compensating: State and Civil Society in Response to Victims of the Armed Conflict in the Ixil Region (Guatemala)," *Human Remains and Violence: An Interdisciplinary Journal* 2, no. 2 (2016).

34 **funerals to be among the most stable:** Peter Brown, *The Cult of the Saints: Its Rise and Function in Latin Christianity* (University of Chicago Press, 2014), 24; Lewis R. Binford, "Mortuary Practices: Their Study and Their Potential," *Memoirs of the Society for American Archaeology* 25 (1971).

34 **The ways of the dead:** See Thomas W. Laqueur, *The Work of the Dead: A Cultural History of Mortal Remains* (Princeton University Press, 2015), 93.

34 **catastrophic violence can bring:** Gila S. Silverman, Aurélien Baroiller, and Susan R. Hemer, "Culture and Grief: Ethnographic Perspectives on Ritual, Relationships and Remembering," *Death Studies* 45, no. 1 (2021).

34 **Civil War changed American funerals:** Drew Gilpin Faust, *This Republic of Suffering: Death and the American Civil War* (Vintage Books, 2009).

35 **thoughts like these:** Many in the field have asked similar questions. See, for example, Ryan Cecil Jobson, "The Case for Letting Anthropology Burn: Sociocultural Anthropology in 2019," *American Anthropologist* 122, no. 2 (2020).

35 **Memory is a battleground:** Elizabeth A. Oglesby and Diane M. Nelson, eds., *Guatemala, the Question of Genocide* (Routledge, 2018).

35 **NO HUBO GENOCIDIO:** Virginia Garrard-Burnett, "Living with Ghosts: Death, Exhumation, and Reburial Among the Maya in Guatemala," *Latin American Perspectives* 42, no. 3 (2015): 189.

36 **Is this doing more harm than good:** For an in-depth exploration of the benefits and limitations of psychosocial accompaniment, including discussions of retraumatization, see Perez-Sales and Navarro Garcia, *Resistencias Contra el Olvido*.

39 **complex patterns of Ixil Maya weaving:** María Luz García, "Discourse, Social Cohesion and the Politics of Historical Memory in the Ixhil Maya Region of Guatemala" (PhD diss., University of Texas at Austin, 2012), 52.

39 **"They had no clothes":** Ibid., 48.

39 **An ancient form of expressing grief:** Lament is a vast topic, but

works that have influenced my thinking include Charles L. Briggs, "'Since I Am a Woman, I Will Chastise My Relatives': Gender, Reported Speech, and the (Re)production of Social Relations in Warao Ritual Wailing," *American Ethnologist* 19, no. 2 (1992); Charles L. Briggs and Clara Mantini-Briggs, *Tell Me Why My Children Died: Rabies, Indigenous Knowledge, and Communicative Justice* (Duke University Press, 2016); Veena Das, *Life and Words: Violence and the Descent into the Ordinary* (University of California Press, 2006); Nadia Seremetakis, *The Last Word: Women, Death, and Divination in Inner Mani* (University of Chicago Press, 1991); Ann Suter, ed., *Lament: Studies in the Ancient Mediterranean and Beyond* (Oxford University Press, 2008).

39   **"to honour and appease the dead":** Margaret Alexiou, *The Ritual Lament in Greek Tradition* (Rowman and Littlefield, 2002), 3.

Chapter 3: Día de los Muertos

41   **A pirate funeral industry:** Associated Press, "Guatemalan Funeral Homes Compete for Corpses," *The San Diego Union Tribune*, November 29, 2009; Lisa Mullins and Jill Replogle, "Crime in Guatemala Boosts Funeral Business," *The World*, May 6, 2009.

45   **"blackened with vultures":** Ricardo Falla, *Negreaba de Zopilotes: Masacre y Sobrevivencia Finca San Francisco, Nentón, 1871–2010* (AVANSCO, 2011).

46   **The cemetery has run out of space:** Jorge Dan Lopez, "Reburying the Dead," Reuters, November 18, 2014; Kevin Lewis O'Neill, "There Is No More Room: Cemeteries, Personhood, and Bare Death," *Ethnography* 13, no. 4 (2012): 524; Henry Pocasangre, "Cementerio General Hará Exhumaciones por Falta de Pago," *Prensa Libre*, February 17, 2017.

46   **A nicho costs:** O'Neill, "There Is No More Room," 524.

46   **In some parts of Guatemala:** The kites of Santiago Sacatepequez and Sumpango and other Guatemalan Day of the Dead traditions are described in María Herrera-Sobek, ed., *Celebrating Latino Folklore: An Encyclopedia of Cultural Traditions* (ABC-CLIO, 2012).

Chapter 4: An Archive of Surveillance

47 **In July 2005, investigators entered:** Kirsten Weld, *Paper Cadavers: The Archives of Dictatorship in Guatemala* (Duke University Press, 2014); Carlos Aguirre and Kate Doyle, *Del Silencio a la Memoria: Revelaciones del Archivo Histórico de la Policía Nacional* (AHPN, 2011). Published in English as *From Silence to Memory: Revelations of the AHPN* (University of Oregon Libraries, 2013).

47 **"staring down a tidal wave":** Ginger Thompson, "Mildewed Police Files May Hold Clues to Atrocities in Guatemala," *The New York Times,* November 21, 2005.

47 **Infested with cockroaches:** Descriptions of the original state of the archive are based on Weld, *Paper Cadavers;* Thompson, "Mildewed Police Files"; Kate Doyle, "The Atrocity Files: Deciphering the Archives of Guatemala's Dirty War," *Harpers,* December 2007.

47 **largest secret cache of state documents:** Weld, *Paper Cadavers,* 2.

48 *One Hundred Years of Solitude:* Gabriel García Márquez, *One Hundred Years of Solitude* (Penguin, 2014).

48 **a giant sinkhole:** Weld, *Paper Cadavers,* 41–42.

48 **The documents are digitally preserved:** Weld, *Paper Cadavers,* 299n34; Josep Fernández Trabal et al., "The Historical Archive of the National Police of Guatemala 2005–2017," Swisspeace, 2021.

48 **attacked with Molotov cocktails:** Weld reports five Molotov attacks. Weld, *Paper Cadavers,* 242.

48 **death threats:** Ibid., 45.

49 **"a kind of micro-chaos":** Rodrigo Rey Rosa, *Human Matter: A Fiction* (University of Texas Press, 2019), 4.

49 **United Fruit Company:** Jason M. Colby, *The Business of Empire: United Fruit, Race, and U.S. Expansion in Central America* (Cornell University Press, 2011); Stephen Kinzer and Stephen Schlesinger, *Bitter Fruit: The Story of the American Coup in Guatemala* (Harvard University Press, 1999).

49 **United States funded and advised:** Hal Brands, *Latin America's Cold War* (Harvard University Press, 2012); Douglas Farah, "Papers Show U.S. Role in Guatemalan Abuses," *The Washington Post,* March 11, 1999; Leslie Gill, *The School of the Americas: Military Training and Political Violence in the Americas* (Duke University Press, 2004); Greg Grandin, *Empire's Workshop: Latin America, the United States, and the Rise of the New Imperialism* (Metropoli-

tan Books, 2006); Peter Kornbluh and Kate Doyle, "CIA and Assassinations: The Guatemala 1954 Documents," *National Security Archive Electronic Briefing Book* no. 4 (1994); Richard F. Nyrop, *Guatemala: A Country Study* (United States: Headquarters, Department of the Army, 1984).

49　**"eventually be known as the School":** Garrard-Burnett, *Terror in the Land of the Holy Spirit,* 55. Many members of the Guatemalan military high command studied at SOA (renamed the Western Hemisphere Institute for Security Cooperation in 2001). See Gill, *School of the Americas,* 121; SOA Watch database of School of the Americas graduates.

49　**Fort Bragg, North Carolina:** Garrard-Burnett, *Terror in the Land of the Holy Spirit,* 55.

49　**Inter-American Defense College:** Kathryn Sikkink, *Mixed Signals: U.S. Human Rights Policy and Latin America* (Cornell University Press, 2018), 167.

49　**He became an Evangelical preacher:** Garrard-Burnett, *Terror in the Land of the Holy Spirit,* 55–56.

49　**praised by Ronald Reagan:** Sikkink, *Mixed Signals,* 168.

49　**admired by Pat Robertson:** Garrard-Burnett, *Terror in the Land of the Holy Spirit,* 76, 161.

50　**plans like "Fusiles y Frijoles":** Garrard-Burnett, *Terror in the Land of the Holy Spirit,* 19–20; Jennifer Schirmer, *The Guatemalan Military Project: A Violence Called Democracy* (University of Pennsylvania Press, 1998), 28.

50　**more than ten thousand people:** Amnesty International, *Guatemala.*

50　**"drain the water":** "quitar al agua del pes." Sanford, *Buried Secrets,* 154–55.

50　**violence in Guatemala as genocide:** Oglesby and Nelson, *Guatemala, the Question of Genocide.*

50　**faced little consequence:** Raúl Molina Mejía, "The Struggle Against Impunity in Guatemala," *Social Justice* 26, no. 4 (1999); Nathanael Heasley et al., "Impunity in Guatemala: The State's Failure to Provide Justice in the Massacre Cases," *American University International Law Review* 16 (2000): 1115.

50　**overturned the conviction:** Jo-Marie Burt, "From Heaven to Hell in Ten Days: The Genocide Trial in Guatemala," *Journal of Genocide Research* 18, nos. 2–3 (2016).

51　**"the epicenter of the search":** Erica Henderson, Catherine

Nolin, and Fredy Peccerelli, "Dignifying a Bare Life and Making Place Through Exhumation: Coban CREOMPAZ Former Military Garrison, Guatemala," *Journal of Latin American Geography* (2014): 106.

51 **"FAFG case #1200–2776":** Appears in Diane M. Nelson, *Who Counts?: The Mathematics of Death and Life After Genocide* (Duke University Press, 2015), 68–69.

52 **National Police undertook campaigns:** Weld, *Paper Cadavers;* Aguirre and Doyle, *Del Silencio.*

52 **clandestine detention center:** Weld, *Paper Cadavers,* 2.

52 **"disappearance" was coined:** Erica Henderson, "Seeking Justice in Guatemala: Dignifying the 'Disappeared' in a Context of Impunity" (thesis, University of Northern British Columbia, 2017), 47; Amnesty International, *"Disappearances": A Workbook,* 1981.

52 **Nacht und Nebel:** Tullio Scovazzi and Gabriella Citroni, *The Struggle Against Enforced Disappearance and the 2007 United Nations Convention* (Martinus Nijhoff, 2007), 4.

52 **"vanish without leaving a trace":** Ibid.

53 **"uncertain as to the fate":** Regulations signed by Field Marshal Wilhelm Keitel on December 12, 1941. Ibid., 5.

53 **innovation in war crimes:** Ibid., 4.

53 **recognized as a crime against humanity:** Ibid., 255.

53 **"They took away our right to life":** He wrote an article on this topic: Alberto Fuentes-Rosales, "In Guatemala, They Stripped Us of the Right to Life, but Also the Right to Die," *Temas de Nuestra América Revista de Estudios Latinoaméricanos* 33, no. 61 (2017).

53 **folder labeled "Myrna Mack Chang":** Kate Doyle, "The Guatemalan Police Archives," *National Security Archive Electronic Briefing Book* No. 170, November 21, 2005.

53 **"Talented, spirited, and audacious":** Elizabeth Oglesby, "Myrna Mack," in *Fieldwork Under Fire: Contemporary Studies of Violence and Survival,* eds. Carolyn Nordstrom and Antonius C.G.M. Robben (University of California Press, 1995), 254. Myrna Mack's 1990 research team included two U.S. researchers (Paula Worby and Elizabeth Oglesby) and a Guatemalan researcher (Rubio Caballeros). Thank you to Elizabeth Oglesby for calling this to my attention.

54 **"destroyed an entire fleet":** Ibid., 255.

54 **among the first Guatemalan researchers:** Americas Watch Committee and Physicians for Human Rights, *Guatemala: Getting*

Away with Murder (Human Rights Watch Publications, 1991), 40. Myrna Mack's mentors were Guatemalan anthropologists Joaquín Noval and Ricardo Falla, a Jesuit priest who documented state violence against Maya communities and their resistance and was forced into exile. Writing in 2000, anthropologist Jeffrey A. Sluka recounted: "The three leading Guatemalan anthropologists have been Victor Montejo, Myrna Mack, and Ricardo Falla. As a result of their research, Montejo, a Mayan, was forced into exile in 1982, Mack was brutally assassinated by a soldier in 1990, and Falla lives in exile after being threatened by the Guatemalan army in 1992. Among the anthropologists who have worked in Guatemala, there is a strong sense of commitment and purpose, and some of them have literally been prepared to die for it." Jeffrey A. Sluka, "Introduction: State Terror and Anthropology," in *Death Squad: The Anthropology of State Terror,* ed. Jeffrey A. Sluka (University of Pennsylvania Press, 2000). See Joaquín Noval, *Resumen Etnográfico de Guatemala* (Editorial Universitaria, 1967); Ricardo Falla, *Massacres in the Jungle: Ixcan, Guatemala, 1975–1982* (Taylor and Francis, 2021); Ricardo Falla, *Quiché Rebelde: Religious Conversion, Politics, and Ethnic Identity in Guatemala* (University of Texas Press, 2014).

54 **"She knew the risks"**: Elizabeth Oglesby, "An Arc Bent Toward Justice: How Myrna Mack's Research Helped Prove Genocide in Guatemala Decades After Her Murder," *LASA Forum* 51, no. 1 (2020): 26.

54 **"The difference between a U.S. scholar"**: Oglesby, "Myrna Mack," 255.

54 **"love-hate" relationship**: Manz, *Paradise in Ashes,* 13.

54 **"ceremonial exchanges, Saint's Day rituals"**: Orin Starn, "Missing the Revolution: Anthropologists and the War in Peru," in *Rereading Cultural Anthropology,* ed. George E. Marcus (Duke University Press, 1992), 168.

54 **"diverted its gaze"**: Linda Green discusses what she calls "anthropology's diverted gaze," concluding that "what is at stake are the struggles between the powerful and the powerless, and what is at issue for anthropologists is to decide with whom to cast their lot." Linda Green, *Fear as a Way of Life: Mayan Widows in Rural Guatemala* (Columbia University Press, 1999), 58.

54 **"What troubles me"**: From a letter written by Myrna Mack dated May 29, 1988, cited in Oglesby, "Myrna Mack," 256.

54 **"I still wonder how":** From a letter written by Myrna Mack dated June 24, 1988, cited in ibid., 256–57.

55 **"I have seen new places":** From a letter written by Myrna Mack dated April 7, 1989, cited in ibid., 258.

55 **"They killed Myrna last night":** Oglesby, "Myrna Mack," 254.

55 **"didn't want to work":** Quoted in Cindy Forster, "Myrna Mack, a Guatemalan Hero," *Against the Current* no. 103 (March/April 2003).

56 **relentlessly sought justice:** David Baluarte and Erin Chlopak, "The Case of Myrna Mack Chang: Overcoming Institutional Impunity in Guatemala," *Human Rights Brief* 10, no. 3 (2003): 19; Americas Watch Committee and Physicians for Human Rights, "Guatemala: Getting Away with Murder" (Human Rights Watch Publications, 1991). See also Inter-American Court of Human Rights, *Case of Myrna Mack Chang v. Guatemala*, Judgment of November 25, 2003; Elise Cossart-Daly, "Myrna Mack Chang vs Guatemala Case Summary," *Loyola of Los Angeles International and Comparative Law Review* 36 (2014).

56 **it "backfired":** Americas Watch Committee and Physicians for Human Rights, "Guatemala: Getting Away with Murder," 41.

56 **Decades after its initial publication:** Oglesby, "An Arc Bent Toward Justice."

56 **"living and combatiente legacy":** Nelson, *Reckoning*, xxxiii. See also ibid., 56–57.

56 **Hannah Arendt famously described:** Hannah Arendt, *Eichmann in Jerusalem: A Report on the Banality of Evil* (Penguin, 1963).

56 **Vucetich system:** Doyle, "The Atrocity Files," 62; Julia Rodriguez, "South Atlantic Crossings: Fingerprints, Science, and the State in Turn-of-the-Century Argentina," *The American Historical Review* 109, no. 2 (2004).

56 **under the supervision of the United States:** Weld, *Paper Cadavers*, 111–12.

57 **Henry classification system:** Manpreet Singh Dhillon, "Pre-History of DNA: Fingerprinting in India," *Research Journal of Humanities and Social Sciences* 10, no. 3 (2019); Doyle, "The Atrocity Files," 62.

57 **hotels sent their guest registries:** Weld, *Paper Cadavers*, 97.

57 **cameras provided by the U.S.:** Aguirre and Doyle, *From Silence to Memory*, 113–14.

57 **"valuable help":** Ibid., 115.

57 **"arms, ammunition, tear gas":** Ibid.

57 **fingerprinting was no longer reserved:** Ibid., 10, 231.

57 **record state death squads:** Aguirre and Doyle, *From Silence to Memory*; Weld, *Paper Cadavers*.

57 **"Policing is":** Weld, *Paper Cadavers*, 14.

57 **"The work of policing":** Ibid.

57 **Archives are tools and weapons:** For the many ways that archives are used as both, see Jens Boel, Perrine Canavaggio, and Antonio González Quintana, eds., *Archives and Human Rights* (Routledge, 2021).

57 **skin stapled to the paper:** Weld, *Paper Cadavers*, 74.

57 **"dried rose petals":** Rey Rosa, *Human Matter*, 24.

57 **"The same state":** Equipo Argentino de Antropología Forense, *Annual Report 2003* (EAAF, 2003), 22. See also César Tcach Abed, "The End of Negationism in Latin America: The Argentine Forensic Anthropology Team," in *Forensic Anthropology Teams in Latin America*, ed. Silvia Dutrénit-Bielous (Routledge, 2019).

58 **"There is no political power":** Jacques Derrida, *Archive Fever: A Freudian Impression* (University of Chicago Press, 1996), 4.

58 **relevant files had been lost:** Kirsten Weld, "Chronicle of a Backlash Foretold: Guatemala's National Police Archives, Lost and Found and Lost—and Found?—Again," in *Archives and Human Rights*, 311.

58 **when the junta left power:** CONADEP, *Nunca Más: The Report of the Argentine National Commission on the Disappeared* (Farrar, Straus and Giroux, 1986), 263–64; Mariana Nazar, "Archives for Truth and Justice in Argentina: The Search for the Missing Persons," in *Archives and Human Rights*, 299.

58 **"piñata of self-forgiveness":** Francisco Goldman, *The Art of Political Murder: Who Killed Bishop Gerardi?* (Atlantic Books, 2010), 13.

58 **systematic attack:** Weld, "Chronicle of a Backlash"; Cora Currier, "A Vast Archive Exposed the Secret History of Kidnapping and Assassination in Guatemala. Now It's Under Threat," *The Intercept*, June 8, 2019.

59 **When the archive was closed:** Weld, "Chronicle of a Backlash," 313.

59 **The "history of the techniques":** Eyal Weizman, *Forensis: The Architecture of Public Truth* (Sternberg, 2014), 11.

59 **Surveillance expands:** See Steven Feldstein, "The Global Expansion of AI Surveillance," Carnegie Endowment for International

Peace, 2019; "Urgent Action Needed Over Artificial Intelligence Risks to Human Rights," United Nations News, September 15, 2021.

Chapter 5: Teaching Skeleton

60 **systems of classification:** See, for example, Steven N. Byers, *Introduction to Forensic Anthropology* (Taylor and Francis, 2016), 30–54; Lee Meadows Jantz, "Skeletal Examination and Documentation," in *Forensic Anthropology: A Comprehensive Introduction*, eds. Natalie R. Langley and MariaTeresa A. Tersigni-Tarrant (CRC Press, 2017).

61 **What will happen to these bodies:** For an account of how one community chose to bury unidentified remains, see Nina Strochlic, "The Cold Cases of Guatemala's Civil War Were Impossible to Identify—Until Now," *National Geographic,* December 19, 2019.

62 **leading to the identification:** Corey Kilgannon, "'Reopening Old Wounds': When 9/11 Remains Are Identified, 20 Years Later," *The New York Times,* September 6, 2021.

62 **consistently retests:** Ibid. See also Jay D. Aronson, *Who Owns the Dead?* (Harvard University Press, 2016); Victor Toom, "Whose Body Is It? Technolegal Materialization of Victims' Bodies and Remains After the World Trade Center Terrorist Attacks," *Science, Technology and Human Values* 41, no. 4 (2016).

62 **"whatever it takes":** Dr. Barbara Sampson, chief medical examiner of New York City, quoted in Kilgannon, "'Reopening Old Wounds.'"

62 **victims' remains are stored:** Luis Fondebrider describes "a common scenario" when "unidentified remains are put into storage indefinitely at a forensic institution, with no further attempt to identify them." Luis Fondebrider, "Reflections on the Scientific Documentation of Human Rights Violations," *International Review of the Red Cross* 84, no. 848 (2002): 889. See also Justin Z. Goldstein et al., "Humanitarian Action in Academic Institutions: A Case Study in the Ethical Stewardship of Unidentified Forensic Cases," *Forensic Sciences Research* (2022).

63 **"major medical schools used slave corpses":** Daina Ramey Berry, *The Price for Their Pound of Flesh: The Value of the Enslaved, from Womb to Grave, in the Building of a Nation* (Beacon Press, 2017); see also Edward C. Halperin, "The Poor, the Black,

and the Marginalized as the Source of Cadavers in United States Anatomical Education," *Clinical Anatomy: The Official Journal of the American Association of Clinical Anatomists and the British Association of Clinical Anatomists* 20, no. 5 (2007): 489–95.

63 *Pernkopf Atlas:* Keiligh Baker, "Eduard Pernkopf: The Nazi Book of Anatomy Still Used by Surgeons," BBC News, August 18, 2019; Sabine Hildebrandt, "How the Pernkopf Controversy Facilitated a Historical and Ethical Analysis of the Anatomical Sciences in Austria and Germany: A Recommendation for the Continued Use of the Pernkopf Atlas," *Clinical Anatomy* 19, no. 2 (2006); Andrew Yee et al., "Ethical Considerations in the Use of Pernkopf's Atlas of Anatomy: A Surgical Case Study," *Surgery* 165, no. 5 (2019).

63 **University of California, Berkeley:** UC Berkeley sits on the ancestral and unceded land of the Chochenyo-speaking Ohlone people, successors of the historic and sovereign Verona Band of Alameda County. For more information, see "Berkeley Sits on Ohlone Land," University of California, Berkeley, Native American Student Development (undated living document).

64 **one of the largest collections:** Sage Alexander, "Grave Robbing at UC Berkeley: A History of Failed Repatriation," *The Daily Californian,* December 5, 2020; Sam Lefebvre, "UC Berkeley Has Only Returned 20% of Its Native American Artifacts and Remains," *Hyperallergic,* June 17, 2020; Richard C. Paddock, "Native Americans Say Berkeley Is No Place for Their Ancestors," *Los Angeles Times,* January 13, 2008.

64 **Hearst Memorial Gymnasium swimming pool:** Paddock, "Native Americans Say Berkeley Is No Place for Their Ancestors." For more recent and detailed information, see Andrew Garrett et al., "Native American Collections in Archives, Libraries, and Museums at the University of California, Berkeley," Working Group Report, Office for the Vice Chancellor of Research, University of California, Berkeley, March 15, 2019.

64 **more than ten thousand individuals:** "Berkeley Talks Transcript: Linda Rugg on Native American Repatriation at UC Berkeley," *Berkeley News,* July 2, 2021. For more on the genocide in California, see Benjamin Madley, *An American Genocide: The United States and the California Indian Catastrophe, 1846–1873* (Yale University Press, 2016).

64 **against the wishes:** Auditor of the State of California, *Native American Graves Protection and Repatriation Act: The Univer-*

sity of California Is Not Adequately Overseeing Its Return of Native American Remains and Artifacts, Report Number: 2019-047, June 11, 2020; Alexander, "Grave Robbing at UC Berkeley: A History of Failed Repatriation"; Lilya Mitelman, "From the Archives: Protesters Call for Return of Relics," *The Daily Californian,* October 8, 2017 (originally published October 8, 2007); Shadi Rahimi, "Senators Accuse UC-Berkeley of Discrimination, Secrecy Over Ancestral Remains," *Indian Country Today,* September 12, 2018.

64 **"We don't appreciate":** Ted Howard, who has since become the chairman of the Shoshone-Paiute Tribes, quoted in Paddock, "Native Americans Say Berkeley Is No Place for Their Ancestors."

64 **remains belonging to children:** Abdul-Aliy A. Muhammad, "Decades After Philadelphia's MOVE Bombing, Penn Museum Still Keeps Secrets on the Remains of 12-Year-Old Girl," *Hyperallergic,* April 20, 2022; Michael Levenson, "Discovery of Bones from MOVE Bombing Jolts Philadelphia Once Again," *The New York Times,* May 15, 2021; Heather Ann Thompson, "Saying Her Name," *The New Yorker,* May 16, 2021. The case is currently being litigated; see Sara Forastieri, "Penn Anthropologist Sues *Inquirer,* Penn, and Others Over Criticism About Her Handling of MOVE Victim Remains," *The Daily Pennsylvanian,* May 26, 2022.

64 **Anthropology is grappling:** The Association of Black Anthropologists (ABA), the Society of Black Archaeologists (SBA), and the Black in Bioanthropology Collective (BiBA), "Collective Statement Concerning the Possession and Unethical Use of Remains," April 28, 2021; Nicholas V. Passalacqua and Marin A. Pilloud, "Unethical Use of 1985 MOVE Bombing Skeletal Remains Highlights Inequality in Death Investigations," *Forensic* (2021); University of Pennsylvania Anthropology Department, "Statement on the MOVE Bombing Human Remains," May 3, 2021; Krystal Strong, "A Requiem for Delisha and Tree Africa," *Anthropology News,* October 25, 2021.

66 **To estimate age at death:** In my fieldwork, "ancestry estimation" was not part of forensic analysis. However, for most forensic anthropologists, it is a standard part of a biological profile, and increasingly debated. For a good overview of debates within the field, see Sabrina Imbler, "Can Skeletons Have a Racial Identity?," *The New York Times,* October 19, 2021.

66 **decision matrices, range charts, indexes:** For more on data analysis, see Byers, *Introduction to Forensic Anthropology,* 18–28.

66 **Standard formulas do not always apply:** Caroline Barker, Ambika Flavel, and Claudia Rivera Fernández, "Forensic Investigations in Guatemala: The Continuing Search for Truth, Justice, and the Missing Two Decades After the Peace Accords," in *Handbook of Forensic Anthropology and Archaeology*, eds. Soren Blau and Douglas H. Ubelaker (Routledge, 2016).

66 **developed from narrow demographic:** Linda L. Klepinger, *Fundamentals of Forensic Anthropology* (John Wiley and Sons, 2006), 81; M. Katherine Spradley et al., "Demographic Change and Forensic Identification: Problems in Metric Identification of Hispanic Skeletons," *Journal of Forensic Sciences* 53, no. 1 (2008).

67 **"For the most part sexual dimorphism":** Natalie R. Langley and MariaTeresa A. Tersigni-Tarrant, eds., *Forensic Anthropology: A Comprehensive Introduction* (CRC Press, 2017), 145.

67 **"In sexing a skull":** Mehmet Yasar Iscan and Maryan Steyn, *The Human Skeleton in Forensic Medicine* (Charles C. Thomas, 2013), 160.

67 **hard physical labor:** K. Krishan and T. Kanchan, "Stature and Build," *Encyclopedia of Forensic Sciences*, eds. Jay A. Siegel, Pekka J. Saukko, and Max M. Houck (Elsevier, 2013).

67 **"populations that may contain smaller":** M. Katherine Spradley, "Metric Methods for the Biological Profile in Forensic Anthropology: Sex, Ancestry, and Stature," *Academic Forensic Pathology* 6, no. 3 (2016): 393; see also Spradley et al., "Demographic Change and Forensic Identification."

67 **Recent research in forensic anthropology:** Sabrina C. Agarwal and Julie K. Wesp, eds., *Exploring Sex and Gender in Bioarchaeology* (University of New Mexico Press, 2017); Evan M. Garofalo and Heather M. Garvin, "The Confusion Between Biological Sex and Gender and Potential Implications of Misinterpretations," in *Sex Estimation of the Human Skeleton*, ed. Alexandra R. Klales (Academic Press, 2020); Stephanie Hartley, Allysha Powanda Winburn, and Itiel E. Dror, "Metric Forensic Anthropology Decisions: Reliability and Biasability of Sectioning-Point-Based Sex Estimates," *Journal of Forensic Sciences* 67, no. 1 (2022); Sean D. Tallman, Caroline D. Kincer, and Eric D. Plemons, "Centering Transgender Individuals in Forensic Anthropology and Expanding Binary Sex Estimation in Casework and Research," *Forensic Anthropology* (2021); Sean D. Tallman, Nicolette M. Parr, and Allysha P. Winburn, "Assumed Differences; Unquestioned Typologies: The Over-

simplification of Race and Ancestry in Forensic Anthropology," *Forensic Anthropology* 4, no. 4 (2021).

67 **culture is written in the body:** Many works explore this theme, such as Thomas Csordas, "Embodiment as a Paradigm for Anthropology," *Ethos* 18, no. 1 (1990); Anne Fausto-Sterling, "The Bare Bones of Sex: Part 1—Sex and Gender," *Signs: Journal of Women in Culture and Society* 30, no. 2 (2005); Clarence C. Gravlee, "How Race Becomes Biology Embodiment of Social Inequality," *American Journal of Physical Anthropology* 139, no. 1 (2009).

68 **proposed by the French sociologist:** Marcel Mauss, *Les Techniques du Corps* (Éditions Payot, 2021). Published in English as Marcel Mauss, "Techniques of the Body," *Economy and Society* 2, no. 1 (1973).

68 **"It was stupid":** Mauss, "Techniques of the Body," 71.

69 **In backstrap weaving:** Carol Hendrickson, *Weaving Identities: Construction of Dress and Self in a Highland Guatemala Town* (University of Texas Press, 1995).

69 **Over time this posture:** Sara K. Becker, "Skeletal Evidence of Craft Production from the Ch'iji Jawira Site in Tiwanaku, Bolivia," *Journal of Archaeological Science: Reports* 9 (2016); Cristian Marcelo Silva Zuñiga, "Exhuming Guatemala's Gender-Based Violence: Justice, Truth-Telling, and Rebuilding in a Post-Conflict Society" (thesis, University of Northern British Columbia, 2011); J. M. Toyne, "Musculoskeletal Stress Markers (MSM) and Weaving Activities at a Prehistoric Coastal Site in Peru," *American Journal of Physical Anthropology* (2003).

69 **"occupational stress markers":** Byers, *Introduction to Forensic Anthropology*, 354–59; Luigi Capasso, Kenneth A. R. Kennedy, and Cynthia A. Wilczak, *Atlas of Occupational Markers on Human Remains* (Edigrafital, 1999); Ana Luísa Santos et al., "The Coimbra Workshop in Musculoskeletal Stress Markers (MSM): An Annotated Review," *Antropologia Portuguesa* 28 (2011).

69 **developing a sort of horn:** David Shahar and Mark G. L. Sayers, "Prominent Exostosis Projecting from the Occipital Squama More Substantial and Prevalent in Young Adult Than Older Age Groups," *Scientific Reports* 8, no. 1 (2018). This study has been critiqued for flaws in methodology; see Denise Grady, "About the Idea That You're Growing Horns from Looking Down at Your Phone . . . ," *The New York Times*, June 20, 2019.

69 **screen time affects our bone mass:** Carmela De Lamas et al.,

"Screen Time and Bone Status in Children and Adolescents: A Systematic Review," *Frontiers in Pediatrics* 9 (2021); Joanne A. McVeigh et al., "Longitudinal Trajectories of Television Watching Across Childhood and Adolescence Predict Bone Mass at Age 20 Years in the Raine Study," *Journal of Bone and Mineral Research* 31, no. 11 (2016).

70 **living bone reacts to force:** Eugénia Cunha and João Pinheiro, "Antemortem Trauma," in *Handbook of Forensic Anthropology and Archaeology*, eds. Soren Blau and Douglas H. Ubelaker (Left Coast Press, 2009).

70 **bone as "green":** Ibid., 322.

71 **The meeting of earth and bone:** Pokines et al., *Manual of Forensic Taphonomy*.

73 **The army arrived in Sepur Zarco:** Alison Crosby and M. Brinton Lykes, *Beyond Repair?: Mayan Women's Protagonism in the Aftermath of Genocidal Harm* (Rutgers University Press, 2019); Susana Navarro García and Paula María Martínez Velázquez, "Psychosocial Work in the Transitional Justice Framework: The Women of Sepur Zarco," in *Human Rights Violations in Latin America: Reparation and Rehabilitation*, eds. Elizabeth Lira, Marcela Cornejo, and Germán Morales (Springer, 2022); Irma A. Velásquez Nimatuj, "The Case of Sepur Zarco and the Challenge to the Colonial State," in *Indigenous Women and Violence: Feminist Activist Research in Heightened States of Injustice*, eds. Lynn Stephen and Shannon Speed (University of Arizona Press, 2021).

73 **list of members of a committee:** Crosby and Lykes, *Beyond Repair?*, 32.

73 **singled out the wives:** Jo-Marie Burt, "Gender Justice in Post-Conflict Guatemala: The Sepur-Zarco Sexual Violence and Sexual Slavery Trial," *Critical Studies* 4 (2019): 67.

73 **Dominga Cuc, was murdered:** Ibid., 80.

74 **"the soldiers' woman":** Crosby and Lykes, *Beyond Repair?*, 74.

74 **"No one asks about you":** Testimony of Petrona Choc Cuc, quoted in Burt, "Gender Justice," 65.

74 **Supported by an alliance:** Asociación de Mujeres Transformando El Mundo, Unión Nacional de Mujeres Guatemaltecas, el Equipo de Estudios Comunitarios y Acción Psicosocial, and Jalok U.

74 **WE ARE ALL SEPUR ZARCO:** Burt, "Gender Justice," 68.

74 **sign of the stigma:** Irma Alicia Velásquez Nimatuj, *"La Justicia Nunca Estuvo de Nuestro Lado": Peritaje Cultural Sobre Conflicto*

Armado y Violencia Sexual en el Caso Sepur Zarco, Guatemala (Hegoa, 2019).

74 **"thorn in the soul":** Crosby and Lykes, *Beyond Repair?*, 74.

74 **the term "muxuk":** Viaene, "Life Is Priceless," 12.

74 **thousands of other women and girls:** Amandine Fulchiron, Olga Alicia Paz, and Angelica Lopez, *Tejidos Que Lleva el Alma: Memoria de Las Mujeres Mayas Sobrevivientes de Violación Sexual Durante el Conflicto Armado* (ECAP, 2009).

74 **Eighty-nine percent of the victims:** CEH, *Memory of Silence*, 54.

75 **Members of the forensic team:** Burt, "Gender Justice," 81.

75 **prayers to protect the souls:** Ibid.

75 **The bones showed bullet wounds:** Ibid.; "En el Juicio del Destacamento Militar Aldea Sepur Zarco, Participan Dos Personas de la FAFG Como Peritus," Fafg.org, October 30, 2020.

75 **the body of Dominga Cuc:** Burt, "Gender Justice," 81.

75 **her daughters were not recovered:** Ibid.

75 **"their bones had turned to dust":** Julia Cuc Choc, quoted in Nina Lakhani, "Justice at Last for Guatemalan Women as Military Officers Jailed for Sexual Slavery," *The Guardian*, March 1, 2016.

76 **"We keep her here with us":** The FAFG continues to have custody of her remains. Her DNA is in the genetic database, but there has been no match to date. Hers are among the many unidentified remains that the team continues to actively attempt to identify through multidisciplinary channels.

76 **The verdict was groundbreaking:** Jo-Marie Burt and Paulo Estrada, "Court Ratifies Historic Sepur Zarco Sexual Violence Judgment," *International Justice Monitor*, July 21, 2017; Whitney Eulich and Louisa Reynolds, "Guatemala War Crimes Verdict Breaks Grip of Impunity," *Christian Science Monitor*, February 26, 2016; Impunity Watch, "Policy Brief: Strategic Litigation for Cases of Sexual and Gender-Based Violence in Guatemala," June 19, 2019; Claudia Martin and Susana SáCouto, "Access to Justice for Victims of Conflict-Related Sexual Violence: Lessons Learned from the Sepur Zarco Case," *Journal of International Criminal Justice* 18, no. 2 (2020); Catalina Ruiz-Navarro, "Guatemala Sexual Slavery Verdict Shows Women's Bodies Are Not Battlefields," *The Guardian*, February 29, 2016.

77 **erupted in cheers:** Burt, "Gender Justice," 68.

Chapter 6: The Ghosts of Argentina

78 **disappearance on a massive scale:** The number of disappeared in Argentina is a matter of politicized debate. Immediately after the dictatorship in 1984, the Argentine truth commission (CONADEP) estimated the number of disappeared at just under nine thousand. Human rights groups put the number at thirty thousand.

78 **"world's first professional war crimes exhumation":** Thomas Keenan and Eyal Weizman, "Mengele's Skull," *Cabinet* 43 (2011).

80 **like the Jorge Luis Borges story:** Jorge Luis Borges, "On Exactitude in Science," in *Collected Fictions*, trans. Andrew Hurley (Penguin, 1999).

81 **Each handwoven huipil is unique:** Barker, Flavel, and Fernández, "Forensic Investigations in Guatemala," 560n28; Carol Hendrickson, *Weaving Identities: Construction of Dress and Self in a Highland Guatemala Town* (University of Texas Press, 1995).

82 **Clothes get switched:** Stefan Schmitt, "Mass Graves and the Collection of Forensic Evidence: Genocide, War Crimes, and Crimes Against Humanity," in *Advances in Forensic Taphonomy: Method, Theory, and Archaeological Perspectives,* eds. William D. Haglund and Marcella H. Sorg (CRC Press, 2001).

82 **find clothing more convincing:** Marta Dillon, *Aparecida* (Sudamericana, 2015); Layla Renshaw, *Exhuming Loss: Memory, Materiality and Mass Graves of the Spanish Civil War* (Left Coast Press, 2011); Sarah E. Wagner, *To Know Where He Lies: DNA Technology and the Search for Srebrenica's Missing* (University of California Press, 2008).

82 **dreams are the primary means:** Garrard-Burnett, "Living with Ghosts; Suazo, *La Cultura Maya ante la Muerte;* Barbara Tedlock, "Quiché Maya Dream Interpretation," *Ethos* 9, no. 4 (1981); Barbara Tedlock, "The Role of Dreams and Visionary Narratives in Mayan Cultural Survival," *Ethos* 20, no. 4 (1992).

82 **"They live, they're not dead":** Suazo, *La Cultura Maya ante la Muerte,* 9.

82 **the dead have needs:** Jean Molesky-Poz, *Contemporary Maya Spirituality: The Ancient Ways Are Not Lost* (University of Texas Press, 2009); Perez-Sales and Navarro Garcia, *Resistencias Contra El Olvido;* Suazo, *La Cultura Maya ante la Muerte.*

82 **"lloran y gritan":** Suazo, *La Cultura Maya ante la Muerte,* 31, 89.

82 **the relationship between them:** As another inhabitant of Rabinal said, "The dead aren't resting and that's why we aren't either, we don't have peace." Suazo, *La Cultura Maya ante la Muerte,* 71.

83 **considered dangerous places:** Zur, *Violent Memories,* 209–11.

83 **communicate through sickness:** Velásquez Nimatuj, *"La Justicia Nunca Estuvo de Nuestro Lado,"* 69.

83 **attributed a measles epidemic:** Zur, *Violent Memories,* 210–11.

83 **In traditional practice:** Barbara Tedlock, "Zuni and Quiche Dream Sharing and Interpretation," in *Dreaming: Anthropological and Psychological Interpretations,* ed. Barbara Tedlock (Cambridge University Press, 1987).

83 **brought survivors dreams:** Garrard-Burnett, "Living with Ghosts"; Tedlock, "The Role of Dreams."

83 **instructing them where to look:** Peccerelli and Henderson, "Forensics and Maya Ceremonies," 312–13; Garrard-Burnett, "Living with Ghosts"; Victoria Aurora Tubin Sotz, "Salud Mental Desde La Perspectiva Maya: Tras La Búsqueda de Una Propuesta a Partir de Las Experiencias de ONG's Que Atienden a las Víctimas del Conflicto Armado en Guatemala" (thesis, Universidad de San Carlos de Guatemala, June 2004); Nimatuj, *"La Justicia Nunca Estuvo de Nuestro Lado."*

83 **"They start talking in dreams":** Rosalina Tuyuc, quoted in Peccerelli and Henderson, "Forensics and Maya Ceremonies," 313.

83 **Isabel was searching:** Garrard-Burnett, "Living with Ghosts," 188–89.

84 **exhumation in a cave:** Suazo, *La Cultura Maya ante la Muerte,* 36.

84 **dream about her missing husband:** Mónica Esmeralda Pinzón González, "Psychosocial Perspectives on the Enforced Disappearance of Indigenous Peoples in Guatemala," in *Missing Persons: Multidisciplinary Perspectives on the Disappeared,* ed. Derek Congram (Canadian Scholars' Press, 2016), 113.

86 **severed Achilles tendon:** Similar evidence has been documented by forensic teams in other mass atrocities, such as the Kibuye massacre in Rwanda. See Danielle Shawn Kurin, *The Bioarchaeology of Disaster: How Catastrophes Change Our Skeletons* (Routledge, 2021), 155, 157.

87 **"The body implies mortality":** Judith Butler, *Precarious Life: The Powers of Mourning and Violence* (Verso Books, 2004), 26.

89 **sleeping in pools of blood:** Nina Strochlic, "The Cold Cases of Guatemala's Civil War Were Impossible to Identify—Until Now," *National Geographic*, December 19, 2019.

89 **skeleton emerged from a closet:** Christopher Joyce and Eric Stover, *Witnesses from the Grave: The Stories Bones Tell* (Ballantine Books, 1992), 304.

89 **Other team members have dreamed:** Courtney Angela Brkic, *The Stone Fields: Love and Death in the Balkans* (Farrar, Straus and Giroux, 2005), 254, 270; Clea Koff, *The Bone Woman: A Forensic Anthropologist's Search for Truth in the Mass Graves of Rwanda, Bosnia, Croatia, and Kosovo* (Random House, 2007), 52.

90 **"It's stupid but I feel like":** Mercedes Salado, quoted in Leila Guerriero, "El Rastro en los Huesos," *Revista Gatopardo* no. 88 (April 2008).

90 **caring for the dead:** For a sensitive and sustained consideration of this theme, see Adam Rosenblatt, "Chapter Five: Caring for the Dead," in *Digging for the Disappeared* (Stanford University Press, 2015).

92 **"multistable perception":** Alexander Pastukhov, "Multistable Perception," in *Oxford Research Encyclopedia of Psychology*, ed. Oliver Braddick (Oxford University Press, 2021).

92 **visual and auditory hallucination:** See, for example, Tanya M. Luhrmann, "Hallucinations and Sensory Overrides," *Annual Review of Anthropology* 40, no. 1 (2011).

Chapter 7: Tucumán Is Burning

94 **"What words":** Marguerite Feitlowitz, *A Lexicon of Terror: Argentina and the Legacies of Torture* (Oxford University Press, 2011), 56.

94 **"The first thing they told me":** Javier Alvarez, quoted in ibid., 59.

95 **He later taught military intelligence:** Martin A. Miller, *The Foundations of Modern Terrorism: State, Society and the Dynamics of Political Violence* (Cambridge University Press, 2013), 210; Luis Roniger, "US Hemispheric Hegemony and the Descent into Genocidal Practices in Latin America," in *State Violence and Genocide in Latin America: The Cold War Years*, eds. Marcia Esparza, Daniel Feierstein, and Henry R. Huttenbach (Routledge, 2009), 38; María Seoane and Vicente Muleiro, *El Dictador: La Historia Secreta y Pública de Jorge Rafael Videla* (Sudamericana, 2012).

95 **"licensed sadism":** Ronald Dworkin, "Introduction," CONADEP, *Nunca Más: The Report of the Argentine National Commission on the Disappeared* (Farrar, Straus and Giroux, 1986), xi.

95 **plan to restructure:** Junta Militar, *Documentos Básicos y Bases Políticas de las Fuerzas Armadas para el Proceso de Reorganización Nacional* (Imprenta del Congreso de la Nación, 1980).

95 **to bring about a "profound transformation":** Feitlowitz, *Lexicon of Terror,* 21.

95 **Spanish title:** Franz Kafka, *El Proceso* (Ediciones Colihue, 2006).

96 **"common sense disinclination":** Hannah Arendt, *The Origins of Totalitarianism* (Harcourt Brace Jovanovich, 1979), 437.

96 **"the energetic protection of human rights":** Videla, quoted in Jo Fisher, *Mothers of the Disappeared* (South End Press, 1989), 12.

96 **"The ideal subject of totalitarian rule":** Arendt, *Origins of Totalitarianism,* 474.

96 **the opera and popular magazines:** "Officers replaced civilians . . . even as director of Buenos Aires' famous opera house, the Téatro Colon." Thomas C. Wright, *State Terrorism in Latin America: Chile, Argentina, and International Human Rights* (Rowman and Littlefield, 2006), 101. "The entire Atlántida publishing group, which owned *Somos* and *Gente,* as well as *Para Tí,* was coopted by the regime." Feitlowitz, *Lexicon of Terror,* 54n79.

96 **New York public relations firm:** Feitlowitz, *Lexicon of Terror,* 48; Nicolás Sagaian, "78 World Cup: The Advertising Campaign of Burson-Marsteller," in *Papelitos, 78 Historias Sobre un Mundial en Dictadura* (Memoria Abierta, Royal Embassy of the Netherlands, and Revista NAN, 2018).

96 **"untold natural riches":** Feitlowitz, *Lexicon of Terror,* 50.

96 **Argentina hosted the World Cup:** The junta spent 700 million USD, 10 percent of the national budget, on the World Cup. Frank Graziano, *Divine Violence: Spectacle, Psychosexuality, and Radical Christianity in the Argentine "Dirty War"* (Westview Press, 1992), 122; for more on the 1978 World Cup, see Matías Bauso, *78: Historia Oral del Mundial* (Sudamericana, 2018); Gustavo Veiga, *Deportes, Desaparecidos y Dictadura* (Alarco Ediciones, 2019).

96 **could hear the cheering crowds:** Michael Welch, *The Bastille Effect: Transforming Sites of Political Imprisonment* (University of California Press, 2022), 112.

96 **chupadero (noun):** Feitlowitz, *Lexicon of Terror,* 62 (definition adapted).

96   **chupado/a (noun):** Ibid. (definition adapted).

96   **tratamiento (noun):** Ibid., 68 (definition adapted).

96   **vuelo (noun):** Ibid. (definition adapted).

97   **reeling between dictatorship and democracy:** Ezequiel Ada-movsky, *Historia de la Argentina: Biografía de un País desde la Conquista Española hasta Nuestros Días* (Buenos Aires: Crítica, 2020); David Rock, *Authoritarian Argentina: The Nationalist Movement, Its History, and Its Impact* (University of California Press, 1993); Luis Alberto Romero, *A History of Argentina in the Twentieth Century* (Penn State University Press, 2021).

97   **dominated Argentine politics:** James W. McGuire, *Peronism Without Perón: Unions, Parties, and Democracy in Argentina* (Stanford University Press, 1997).

97   **Perón rose to power:** Adamovsky, *Historia de la Argentina;* Rock, *Authoritarian Argentina;* Romero, *A History of Argentina.*

97   **"chain effect of happiness":** Romero, *A History of Argentina,* 103.

97   **threefold increase in visitors:** Adamovsky, *Historia de la Argentina.*

97   **the Lady of Hope, the Good Fairy:** Evita's many monikers come from Tomás Eloy Martínez, *Santa Evita* (Vintage Books, 1997); Julie Taylor, *Eva Perón: The Myths of a Woman* (University of Chicago Press, 1981); Diana Taylor, *Disappearing Acts: Spectacles of Gender and Nationalism in Argentina's "Dirty War"* (Duke University Press, 1997).

98   **moved toward totalitarianism:** Adamovsky, *Historia de la Argentina;* Rock, *Authoritarian Argentina;* Romero, *A History of Argentina.*

98   **in the city of Córdoba:** James P. Brennan and Mónica B. Gordillo, "Working Class Protest, Popular Revolt, and Urban Insurrection in Argentina: The 1969 Cordobazo," *Journal of Social History* (1994); Antonius C.G.M. Robben, *Political Violence and Trauma in Argentina* (University of Pennsylvania Press, 2011), 48–49.

98   **forbade everything:** Mala Htun, *Sex and the State: Abortion, Divorce, and the Family Under Latin American Dictatorships and Democracies* (Cambridge University Press, 2003); Daniel G. Kres-sel, "The 'Argentine Franco'?: The Regime of Juan Carlos Onganía and Its Ideological Dialogue with Francoist Spain (1966–1970)," *The Americas* 78, no. 1 (2021): 108; Valeria Manzano, *The Age of Youth*

in Argentina: Culture, Politics, and Sexuality from Perón to Videla
(University of North Carolina Press, 2014).

98 **mobilized a guerrilla movement:** Wright, *State Terrorism,* 97;
Romero, *A History of Argentina,* 181.

98 **two important militant factions emerged:** Ibid.

98 **earned his famous nickname:** Jon Lee Anderson, *Che Guevara:
A Revolutionary Life* (Random House, 1997), 124.

99 **deepened his militancy:** Ibid., 157.

99 **The ERP believed:** Daniel Gutman, *Sangre en el Monte: La In-
creíble Aventura del ERP en los Cerros Tucumanos* (Sudamericana, 2012); Pablo A. Pozzi, *Por las Sendas Argentinas: El PRT-ERP,
la Guerrilla Marxista* (Imago Mundi, 2004).

99 **hotbed of guerrilla activity:** Gutman, *Sangre en el Monte.*

99 **"Tucumán arde":** The phrase "Tucumán is burning" originated
in a political art movement. Leticia Viviana Albarracín, "Arte
y Política: El Caso del 'Tucumán Arde' (1968–1969)," *Revista
nuestrAmérica* 1, no. 1 (2013).

99 **the Quechua word:** Jack Emory Davis, *The Spanish of Argentina
and Uruguay: An Annotated Bibliography for 1940–1978* (Centre
International de Dialectologie Générale, 1966), 234.

99 **won popular support:** Wright, *State Terrorism,* 97.

99 **"Robin Hood" escapades:** Romero, *A History of Argentina,* 190.

99 **pallets of soda:** David Cox, *Dirty Secrets, Dirty War: Buenos Aires,
Argentina, 1976–1983: The Exile of Editor Robert J. Cox* (Evening
Post Books, 2008), 47.

99 **"marked the guerrilla organizations' official birth":** Romero,
A History of Argentina, 189; see also Robben, *Political Violence
and Trauma,* 107–9, 112–15.

100 **the exiled Perón's influence grew:** Romero, *A History of Argentina,* 186.

100 **political image with broad appeal:** Ernesto Laclau, *On Populist
Reason* (Verso Books, 2018), 220; Robben, *Political Violence and
Trauma,* 66; Wright, *State Terrorism,* 98.

100 **a deadly gun battle:** Robben, *Political Violence and Trauma,*
65–70.

101 **submarino (noun):** Feitlowitz, *Lexicon of Terror,* 67–68 (definition
adapted).

101 **Several of the secret torture centers:** CONADEP, *Nunca Más,*
102, 103, 200.

101 **"Marxists, subversives, and terrorists":** Gustavo Morello, SJ, *The Catholic Church and Argentina's Dirty War* (Oxford University Press, 2015), 61.

102 **"If Evita were alive":** Rock, *Authoritarian Argentina*, 218.

102 *Evita Montonera:* Robben, *Political Violence and Trauma*, 266.

102 **first woman in the world:** There were earlier female heads of state, such as Sirima Ratwatte Dias Bandaranaike, who became the prime minister of Sri Lanka in 1960.

102 **first-ever union strike:** McGuire, *Peronism Without Perón*, 167.

102 **"There is only one Evita":** Mirta Zaida Lobato, María Damilakou, and Lizel Tornay, "Working-Class Beauty Queens Under Peronism," in *The New Cultural History of Peronism: Power and Identity in Mid-Twentieth-Century Argentina*, eds. Matthew B. Karush and Oscar Chamosa (Duke University Press, 2010), 193.

102 **"hysterical and out-of-control":** Taylor, *Disappearing Acts*, 54.

102 **"visibly deteriorated":** Videla, quoted in ibid., 55.

102 **Alianza Anticomunista Argentina:** Robben, *Political Violence and Trauma*, 136–38.

102 **He first unleashed:** Ibid., 138.

102 **"to neutralize and/or annihilate the activities":** Ibid., 149n3.

103 **the already weakened ERP:** Robben, *Political Violence and Trauma*, 173; Wright, *State Terrorism*, 100; James P. Brennan, *Argentina's Missing Bones: Revisiting the History of the Dirty War* (University of California Press, 2018), 40.

103 **"testing ground":** Daniel Feierstein, *Genocide as Social Practice: Reorganizing Society Under the Nazis and Argentina's Military Juntas* (Rutgers University Press, 2014), 132. See also Anita Jemio, "El Operativo Independencia en el Sur Tucumano (1975–1976): Las Formas de la Violencia Estatal en los Inicios del Genocidio" (PhD diss., Universidad de Buenos Aires, 2010).

103 **the genocide had begun:** Romero, *A History of Argentina*, 213.

105 **"The entire nation responded with relief":** Quoted in Patricia M. Marchak, *God's Assassins: State Terrorism in Argentina in the 1970s* (McGill-Queen's University Press, 1999), 212.

105 **"Now we are governed by gentlemen":** Quoted in Rita Arditti, *Searching for Life: The Grandmothers of the Plaza de Mayo and the Disappeared Children of Argentina* (University of California Press, 1999), 8. Borges later spoke out against the dictatorship: see Arditti, *Searching for Life*, 40; Feitlowitz, *Lexicon of Terror*, 7n12;

Lawrence Weschler, *A Miracle, A Universe: Settling Accounts with Torturers* (University of Chicago Press, 1998), 18.

105 **lists of clandestine detention centers:** Secretaría de Derechos Humanos de la Nación, "Anexo V: Listado de Centros Clandestinos de Detención y Otros Lugares de Reclusión Ilegal del Terrorismo de Estado En La Argentina Entre 1974 y 1983," in *Registro Unificado de Víctimas del Terrorismo de Estado*, Ministerio de Justicia y Derechos Humanos de La Nación, July 2015.

105 **eight hundred clandestine centers identified:** Secretaría de Derechos Humanos de la Nación, "Sitios y Espacios de Memoria," August 30, 2017.

105 **The first was La Escuelita de Famaillá:** CONADEP, *Nunca Más*, 198.

106 **a battery-operated field telephone:** Ibid., 198–99.

106 **"In drawing up this report":** Ibid., 20.

106 **soldiers tied red bands:** Ibid., 199.

106 **a prisoner buried alive:** Ibid., 202.

106 **one of the largest mass graves:** Víctor Ataliva et al., "Arqueología Forense Desde las Profundidades: Pozo de Vargas, Tucumán (2002–2019): Una Síntesis," in *Arqueología Forense y Procesos de Memorias: Saberes y Reflexiones Desde las Practices,* eds. Víctor Ataliva, Aldo Gerónimo, and Ruy D. Zurita (Universidad Nacional de Tucumán, 2019).

107 **El Colectivo de Arqueología:** Until 2009, the team was known as Grupo Interdisciplinario de Arqueología y Antropología de Tucumán (GIAAT); for simplicity I use CAMIT throughout.

107 **archaeologists began meeting:** Ataliva et al., "Arqueología Forense Desde las Profundidades"; see also Fernando Ávila and Nacho Sacaluga, dirs., *Noche del Mundo* (Universidad Europea, Fundación Inquietarte, 2016).

108 **parrilla (noun):** Feitlowitz, *Lexicon of Terror,* 56 (definition adapted).

108 **asado (noun):** Ibid., 61 (definition adapted).

109 **"First we will kill":** Ibérico Saint Jean, governor of the Province of Buenos Aires, May 1976; Federico Finchelstein, *The Ideological Origins of the Dirty War: Fascism, Populism, and Dictatorship in Twentieth Century Argentina* (Oxford University Press, 2017), 127.

109 **"Just as this fire now destroys":** Feitlowitz, *Lexicon of Terror,* 186n32.

109 **"A terrorist is not only":** CONADEP, *Nunca Más,* 333.

109 **People were disappeared because:** Ibid., 60–61.

109 **Indigenous communities:** Víctor Ataliva and Patricia Arenas, "Comunidades Indígenas y Prácticas Sociales Genocidas en Tucumán (1975–1983): Apuntes Para un Diagnóstico," in Ataliva, Gerónimo, and Zurita, eds., *Arqueología Forense y Procesos de Memorias;* Diana Isabel Lenton, "De Genocidio en Genocidio: Notas Sobre el Registro de La Represión a La Militancia Indígena," *Revista de Estudios Sobre Genocidio* 13 (2018); Gastón Gordillo and Silvia Hirsch, "Indigenous Struggles and Contested Identities in Argentina Histories of Invisibilization and Reemergence," *Journal of Latin American Anthropology* 8, no. 3 (2003).

109 **Jewish Argentines:** Emmanuel Nicolás Kahan, *Memories That Lie a Little: Jewish Experiences During the Argentine Dictatorship,* trans. David Foster (Brill, 2019). For personal accounts, see Alicia Partnoy, *The Little School: Tales of Disappearance and Survival,* trans. Alicia Partnoy, with Lois Athey and Sandra Braunstein (Midnight Editions, 1998); Nora Strejilevich, *A Single Numberless Death,* trans. Cristina de la Torre, with collaboration of author (University of Virginia Press, 2002); Jacobo Timerman, *Prisoner Without a Name, Cell Without a Number,* trans. Toby Talbot (Vintage Books, 1981).

110 **widespread anti-Semitism:** Finchelstein, *Ideological Origins of the Dirty War,* 135–43; Marisa Braylan et al., *Report on the Situation of the Jewish Detainees-Disappeared During the Genocide Perpetrated in Argentina* (Social Research Center of Argentinean Jewish Community Centers Association, 2000).

110 **Nazi sympathies:** CONADEP, *Nunca Más,* 67–72; Feitlowitz, *Lexicon of Terror,* 92; Finchelstein, *Ideological Origins of the Dirty War,* 135–43; Morello, *Catholic Church and Argentina's Dirty War,* 26–27.

110 **painted with swastikas:** Cox, *Dirty Secrets, Dirty War,* 100; Finchelstein, *Ideological Origins of the Dirty War,* 135–43.

110 **Jewish prisoners were singled out:** CONADEP, *Nunca Más,* 67–72.

110 **"How did your military superiors":** Interview between journalist Fernando Almirón and former sergeant Víctor Ibáñez, quoted in Finchelstein, *Ideological Origins of the Dirty War,* 8–9.

110 **"He told me they knew":** Dr. Norberto Liwsky, quoted in CONADEP, *Nunca Más,* 21–22.

111 **The word "genocide":** Donald Bloxham and A. Dirk Moses, eds.,

The Oxford Handbook of Genocide Studies (Oxford University Press, 2010); Raphael Lemkin, "Genocide," *The American Scholar*, April 15, 1946.

111 **"national, ethnical, racial or religious group":** United Nations General Assembly, Convention on the Prevention and Punishment of the Crime of Genocide, Article II, December 9, 1948.

112 **political and social groups:** For more discussion of this theme, see Bloxham and Moses, eds., *Handbook of Genocide Studies;* Feierstein, *Genocide as Social Practice;* Lemkin, "Genocide"; Alexander Laban Hinton, *Annihilating Difference: The Anthropology of Genocide* (University of California Press, 2002).

112 **"Genocide" was used to characterize:** CONADEP, *Nunca Más*, 234; Antonius C.G.M. Robben, "From Dirty War to Genocide: Argentina's Resistance to National Reconciliation," *Memory Studies* 5, no. 3 (2012); Feierstein, *Genocide as Social Practice.*

112 **"Dirty War":** Finchelstein recounts: "The criminal actions of the junta were called the 'Dirty War' by perpetrators, a term which was later used uncritically by its victims and bystanders alike." He writes: "This is a popularized term that needs to be explained in terms of the country's fascist genealogies. From a historical perspective, the Dirty War did not feature two combatants but rather victims and perpetrators." Finchelstein, *Ideological Origins of the Dirty War*, 123, 3. For more on the term's genealogy, see Robben, "From Dirty War to Genocide."

112 **To the encyclopedia of horror:** CONADEP, *Nunca Más*, 20.

112 **The "task forces":** Ibid., 11–13; Romero, *A History of Argentina*, 217–18.

113 **"I categorically deny":** Videla, quoted in Fisher, *Mothers of the Disappeared*, 62.

113 **"because of the uncertainty":** Interamerican Commission on Human Rights, 1977 Report, quoted in Scovazzi and Citroni, *The Struggle Against Enforced Disappearance*, 342.

113 **"You're dirt":** Dr. Norberto Liwsky, quoted in CONADEP, *Nunca Más*, 25.

113 **Exhumation is not just a matter:** For a technical discussion of the exhumation of the Pozo, see Víctor Hugo Ataliva et al., "Arqueología Forense: Aspectos Técnicos y Metodológicos de una Intervención Compleja, Pozo de Vargas (Tucumán, Argentina)," *Revista Internacional de Anthropología y Odontología Forense* 4, no. 2 (April 2021).

Chapter 8: Touching Bones

116   **The team has searched for the disappeared:** Pedro Pérez-Torres and Derek Congram, "Biografía: Equipo Argentino de Antropología Forense (EAAF)," *Forensic Anthropology* 5, no. 3 (2022); Mercedes Salado Puerto, Laura Catelli, Carola Romanini, Magdalena Romero, and Carlos María Vullo, "The Argentine Experience in Forensic Identification of Human Remains," in *Forensic Science and Humanitarian Action: Interacting with the Dead and the Living,* eds. Roberto C. Parra, Sara C. Zapico, and Douglas H. Ubelaker (John Wiley and Sons, 2020).

117   **Before 1984, human rights forensics:** For an excellent overview of the field, see Rosenblatt, *Digging for the Disappeared.*

117   **Heavy machinery clawed:** Patricia Bernardi and Luis Fondebrider, "Forensic Archaeology and the Scientific Documentation of Human Rights Violations: An Argentinean Example from the Early 1980s," in *Forensic Archaeology and Human Rights Violations*, ed. Roxana Ferllini (Charles C. Thomas, 2007); Mercedes Doretti and Clyde C. Snow, "Forensic Anthropology and Human Rights," in *Hard Evidence: Case Studies in Forensic Anthropology*, ed. Dawnie Wolfe Steadman (Routledge, 2016), 526.

118   **The newly formed truth commission:** For a detailed history of CONADEP, see Emilio Crenzel, *The Memory of the Argentina Disappearances: The Political History of Nunca Más* (Routledge, 2012).

118   **Grandmothers of Plaza de Mayo:** Arditti, *Searching for Life.*

118   **"an alternative origin story":** Lindsay Smith, "'Genetics Is a Study in Faith': Forensic DNA, Kinship Analysis, and the Ethics of Care in Post-conflict Latin America," *Scholar & Feminist Online* 11, no. 3 (2013).

118   **Dr. Clyde Snow:** Snow's career, including his work in Argentina, is detailed in Joyce and Stover, *Witnesses from the Grave.*

118   **"They were losing evidence":** Clyde Snow, quoted in Lindsay A. Smith, "The Missing, the Martyred and the Disappeared: Global Networks, Technical Intensification and the End of Human Rights Genetics," *Social Studies of Science* 47, no. 3 (2017): 402.

118   **a single methodical excavation:** Stephen G. Michaud, "Identifying Argentina's Disappeared," *The New York Times*, December 27, 1987.

119   **"I checked all around":** Ibid.

119 **falsified death certificates:** Doretti and Snow, "Forensic Anthropology and Human Rights," 526–27.

119 **dictatorship-era autopsy report:** Abed, "The End of Negationism in Latin America," 64.

119 **"the most experienced team":** Michaud, "Identifying Argentina's Disappeared."

119 **indelibly marked:** In an interview, Patricia Bernardi said, "At first we were very scared, and this has been a very emotional experience for us all. . . . We knew as soon as we started, we would be marked." Ibid.

121 **"We need to acknowledge":** Rosemary Joyce, "Grave Responsibilities: Encountering Human Remains," in *Disturbing Bodies: Perspectives on Forensic Anthropology*, eds. Rosemary Joyce and Zoë Crossland (School for Advanced Research Press, 2015), 173–75.

121 **"sensual geography":** Joanna Sofaer, "Touching the Body: The Living and the Dead in Osteoarchaeology and the Performance Art of Marina Abramović," *Norwegian Archaeological Review* 45, no. 2 (2012), 141.

122 **"a billowy, flat appearance":** Angi M. Christensen, Nicholas V. Passalacqua, and Eric J. Bartelink, *Forensic Anthropology: Current Methods and Practice* (Academic Press, 2019), 336.

122 **"it is notoriously difficult":** Sofaer, "Touching the Body," 140.

122 **sight dominates:** Constance Classen, *Worlds of Sense: Exploring the Senses in History and Across Cultures* (Routledge, 1993); Robert Jütte, *A History of the Senses: From Antiquity to Cyberspace,* trans. James Lynn (Polity Press, 2005); Karen Barad, "On Touching—the Inhuman That Therefore I Am," *Differences* 23, no. 3 (December 1, 2012).

122 **"sensation of touch":** Constance Classen, ed., *The Book of Touch* (Routledge, 2020), 5.

123 **When Clyde Snow and the students:** In telling the story of the team's first exhumation, I draw from my interviews with Luis Fondebrider and the following texts as my primary sources: CLASCO, *Ciencia por la verdad: 35 Años del Equipo de Antropología Forense* (Consejo Latinoamericano de Ciencias Sociale and Universidad Nacional de Quilmes, 2019); Felipe Celesia, *La Muerte es el Olvido* (Paidós, 2019); Luis Fondebrider, "Forensic Archaeology and Anthropology: A Balance Sheet," in *Memories from Darkness: Archaeology of Repression and Resistance in Latin America* (Springer, 2009); Joyce and Stover, *Witnesses from the Grave;*

Mauricio Cohen Salama, *Tumbas Anónimas: Informe Sobre la Identificación de Restos de Víctimas de la Represión Legal* (Catálogos Editora, 1992).

123 **"I always carry it around":** Quoted in Weil, "Clyde Snow."

124 **the political importance:** For a concise discussion of the tensions between political and apolitical approaches to human rights forensics, see Smith, "The Missing, the Martyred and the Disappeared."

125 **distinctive odor:** Boyd B. Dent, Shari L. Forbes, and Barbara H. Stuart, "Review of Human Decomposition Processes in Soil," *Environmental Geology* 45, no. 4 (2004).

125 **remains are potential vectors:** Byers, *Introduction to Forensic Anthropology;* Michael W. Warren, Heather A. Walsh-Haney, and Laurel Freas, eds., *The Forensic Anthropology Laboratory* (CRC Press, 2008).

126 **"ethos of disregard":** Corinne Duhig and Ron Turnbull, "Crime Scene Management and Forensic Anthropology: Observations and Recommendations from the United Kingdom and International Cases," in *Forensic Archaeology and Human Rights Violations,* ed. Roxana Ferllini (Charles C. Thomas, 2007), 97.

126 **traces of DNA:** Max Houck, ed., *Forensic Anthropology* (Elsevier, 2016), 134.

126 **it feels wrong:** Other anthropologists have also noted how sawing and grinding bones for DNA samples can feel counterintuitive or even upsetting. Forensic anthropologist Clea Koff describes watching someone saw out a sample as "shocking." Koff, *Bone Woman,* 53. Social anthropologist Sarah Wagner, observing DNA samples taken from the remains of victims of the Bosnian war, refers to the process as "violence" and says, "The missing person has lost yet again a part of his body." Wagner, *To Know Where He Lies,* 111.

127 **"very gallant little group":** Quoted in U.S. National Library of Medicine, "Making the 'Disappeared' Visible," *Visible Proofs: Forensic Views of the Body,* February 16, 2006.

127 **rudimentary tools:** Ibid.; Jeff Guntzel, "'The Bones Don't Lie': Forensic Anthropologist Clyde Snow Travels Continents to Bring the Crimes of Mass Murderers to Light," *National Catholic Reporter,* July 30, 2004.

128 **"work in the day":** Quoted in ibid.

128 **"Once this kind of thing":** Ibid.

128 **"Morris, give me the spoon":** Ibid. In another account, it is Mimi who says this. Joyce and Stover, *Witnesses from the Grave,* 247.

128 **"That's when I figured":** Ibid.

128 **taking part in the ritual:** Leila Renshaw and others have discussed the "capacity for archaeologists to animate the dead." In Renshaw's case, it is the discovery of cigarette papers in the pocket of a body being exhumed that sparks recognition among the archaeologists who smoke. Renshaw, *Exhuming Loss,* 157. Renshaw notes, and I agree, that this is beautifully captured in Michael Ondaatje's deeply researched fictional account of exhumation: Michael Ondaatje, *Anil's Ghost* (Random House, 2011).

129 **forensic scientists testify:** For a nuanced discussion of forensic evidence, see Zoë Crossland, "Evidential Regimes of Forensic Archaeology," *Annual Review of Anthropology* 42, no. 1 (2013); Zoë Crossland, "Of Clues and Signs: The Dead Body and Its Evidential Traces," *American Anthropologist* 111, no. 1 (2009).

129 **can come into tension:** Tensions between legal needs and the needs of the families have long been explored in forensic literature. See Mimi Doretti and Luis Fondebrider, "Science and Human Rights: Truth, Justice, Reparation and Reconciliation; A Long Way in Third World Countries," in *Archaeologies of the Contemporary Past,* eds. Victor Buchli, Gavin Lucas, and Margaret Cox (Routledge, 2001); Eric Stover and Rachel Shigekane, "The Missing in the Aftermath of War: When Do the Needs of Victims' Families and International War Crimes Tribunals Clash?," *International Review of the Red Cross* 84, no. 848 (2002).

130 **"Argentina's Nuremberg":** For more on the Trial of the Juntas, see Amnesty International, "Argentina: The Military Juntas and Human Rights; Report of the Trial of the Former Junta Members," January 1, 1987; Gabrielle Esparza, "The Trial of the Juntas: Reckoning with State Violence in Argentina," *Not Even Past,* April 7, 2021; Jo Fisher, *Out of the Shadows* (Monthly Review Press, 1993); Carlos Alberto Silva, *El Núremberg Argentino: El Libro del Juicio Testimonios* (Aura, 1986); Paula K. Speck, "The Trial of the Argentine Junta: Responsibilities and Realities," *The University of Miami Inter-American Law Review* 18 (1986).

131 **"the skeleton is its own best witness":** Quoted in Joyce and Stover, *Witnesses from the Grave,* 268.

131 **"all the markings of an execution":** Quoted in Arditti, *Searching for Life,* 75.

131 **"That's tough to do":** Quoted in Don Stewart, "Witness After Death," *Sooner Magazine,* Fall/Winter 1985, 10.

131 **"justice cascade":** Kathryn Sikkink, *The Justice Cascade: How Human Rights Prosecutions Are Changing World Politics* (W. W. Norton, 2011). See also Kathryn Sikkink, "From Pariah State to Global Protagonist: Argentina and the Struggle for International Human Rights," *Latin American Politics and Society* 50, no. 1 (2008).

131 **"It was fairly clinical":** Quoted in Guntzel, "Bones Don't Lie."

132 **formally became the EAAF:** Pérez-Torres and Congram, "Biografía: Equipo Argentino de Antropología Forense."

132 **bring a human touch to the work:** For example, the care and thought EAAF brings to their relationship with families are evident in this passage from the team's annual report: "Over the years, we have learned to be available when relatives of a disappeared person need information, but also to only contact families when we have very precise information to tell or ask them. Sometimes, even a phone call from EAAF can heighten expectations in a way we do not necessarily intend or cannot fulfill. Even in cases where we have made a positive identification, EAAF members try to investigate which member of the family may be the best contact person to communicate the news to the rest of the family." Equipo Argentino de Antropología Forense, *Annual Report 2006* (EAAF 2006), 20.

132 **"We had a relationship":** Quoted in Guerriero, "El Rastro en los Huesos."

132 **"I began to kiss him":** Quoted in Zoë Crossland, "Buried Lives: Forensic Archaeology and the Disappeared in Argentina," *Archaeological Dialogues* 7, no. 2 (2000): 154.

133 **"The first thing I do":** Patricia Bernardi, quoted in Rosenblatt, *Digging for the Disappeared*, 167.

Chapter 9: Mothers

135 **"Where should we meet?":** Quoted in Fisher, *Mothers of the Disappeared*, 28.

136 **Fridays were unlucky:** Ibid., 29.

136 **"We wore flat shoes":** Ibid., 28.

136 **The Madres de Plaza de Mayo learned as they went:** Ibid., 52–70.

137 **"as if rebelling against":** "La Historia de las Madres de Plaza de Mayo: Érase una Vez Catorce Mujeres," *Lavaca*, March 24, 2022.

137 **the only newspaper that regularly reported:** For a detailed account of the *Buenos Aires Herald* during the dictatorship, see Cox, *Dirty Secrets, Dirty War.*

137 **"lessening the prestige":** Cited in Fisher, *Mothers of the Disappeared,* 25.

137 **"As from today it is forbidden":** Fisher, *Mothers of Disappeared,* 25; see also Jerry W. Knudson, "Veil of Silence: The Argentine Press and the Dirty War, 1976–1983," *Latin American Perspectives* 24, no. 6 (1997): 100–101.

137 **The *Buenos Aires Herald* printed:** Knudson, "Veil of Silence," 101.

137 **"subject to detention":** Fisher, *Mothers of the Disappeared,* 25.

137 **Journalists were particular targets:** "Suman 223 Los Periodistas y Trabajadores de la Comunicación Desaparecidos," *La Tinta,* June 18, 2019; Cox, *Dirty Secrets, Dirty War,* 151; CONADEP, *Nunca Más,* 362–68.

137 **"genocide of journalists":** Jacobo Timerman, "The Bodies Counted Are Our Own," *Columbia Journalism Review,* May/June 1980.

137 **the bestselling book:** Timerman, *Prisoner Without a Name, Cell Without a Number.*

138 **"It was an honour to scream":** Quoted in Uki Goñi, "Pope Francis and the Missing Marxist," *The Guardian,* December 11, 2013.

138 **The terror and ambiguity:** Wright, *State Terrorism,* 108–9; Antonius C.G.M. Robben, *Argentina Betrayed: Memory, Mourning, and Accountability* (University of Pennsylvania Press, 2018), 49.

139 **"There are all kinds of people":** U.S. Congress, House Committee on Foreign Affairs, Subcommittee on International Organizations, *Human Rights and the Phenomenon of Disappearances: Hearings Before the Subcommittee on International Organizations of the Committee on Foreign Affairs, House of Representatives, Ninety-sixth Congress, First Session, September 20, 25, and October 18, 1979,* Appendix 17, "Testimony of Ana María Careaga" (U.S. Government Printing Office, 1980), 614.

139 **she performed immaculate tests:** Sergio Rubin and Francesca Ambrogetti, *Pope Francis: Conversations with Jorge Bergoglio: His Life in His Own Words* (Random House, 2013), 14–15.

140 **hide their books:** Rubin and Ambrogetti, *Pope Francis,* 213; Eduardo Anguita and Daniel Cecchini, "'Le Debo Mucho a Esa Mujer': La Amistad del Papa Francisco con una Madre de Plaza de Mayo que Está Desaparecida," *Infobae,* January 30, 2020.

140 **Madres were devoutly religious:** Fisher, *Mothers of the Disappeared*, 53.

140 **"That was the total interview":** Nelly de Bianchi, quoted in Marchak, *God's Assassins*, 197.

140 **"The Catholic Church turned its back":** Ibid.

140 **"a very pretty letter":** Margarita de Oro, quoted in Fisher, *Mothers of the Disappeared*, 57.

140 **messages to Pope John Paul II:** Emilio Mignone, "The Catholic Church, Human Rights and the 'Dirty War' in Argentina," in *Church and Politics in Latin America*, ed. Dermot Keogh (Palgrave Macmillan, 1990), 364.

140 **when the pope visited Argentina:** Ibid.

140 **"web of mediocrity":** Emilio F. Mignone, *Witness to the Truth: The Complicity of Church and Dictatorship in Argentina, 1976–1983* (Orbis Books, 1986), 28.

140 **Luján pilgrimage:** Débora D'Antonio, "Las Madres de Plaza de Mayo y la Apertura de un Camino de Resistencias," *Revista de Estudios Sobre la Cultura Latinoamericana* 2 (2006): 34; Fisher, *Mothers of the Disappeared*, 54.

140 **Azucena Villaflor emerged:** Arditti, *Searching for Life*, 53; Enrique Arrosagaray, *Biografía de Azucena Villaflor: Creadora del Movimiento Madres de Plaza de Mayo* (Editorial Cienflores, 2021).

141 **"That day, Azucena showed me":** Arditti, *Searching for Life*, 53.

141 **A Madre named Dora de Bazze:** Fisher, *Mothers of the Disappeared*, 62.

141 **"Stick it up":** Dora de Bazze is quoted as saying "Stick it up your . . ." in Fisher, *Mothers of the Disappeared*, 62; I have taken the liberty of filling in the omitted word.

142 **commandeer a city bus:** "La Historia de las Madres de Plaza de Mayo."

142 **the mothers would shout:** Fisher, *Mothers of the Disappeared*, 61–62.

142 **"the crazy women":** For more on the gendered dimensions of the Madres' activism, see Marguerite Guzman Bouvard, *Revolutionizing Motherhood: The Mothers of the Plaza de Mayo* (Rowman and Littlefield, 1994); Matilde Mellibovsky, *Circle of Love Over Death: Testimonies of the Mothers of the Plaza de Mayo* (Curbstone Press, 1997); Taylor, *Disappearing Acts*.

142 **"Our children gave birth to us":** For an in-depth examination of this slogan, see Cecilia Sosa, *Queering Acts of Mourning in the Af-*

termath of Argentina's Dictatorship: The Performances of Blood (Boydell & Brewer, 2014).

142 **"the regime's depravity"**: Feitlowitz, *Lexicon of Terror*, 78; see also Miriam Lewin and Olga Wornat, *Putas y Guerrilleras: Crímenes Sexuales en Los Centros Clandestinos de Detención* (Planeta, 2014); Barbara Sutton, *Surviving State Terror: Women's Testimonies of Repression and Resistance in Argentina* (New York University Press, 2018).

142 **alive in a nightmare**: U.S. Congress, "Testimony of Ana María Careaga," 615.

143 **"I could hear people"**: Ana María Careaga, quoted in Feitlowitz, *Lexicon of Terror*, 60.

143 **"We were in the world"**: Ibid., 193.

143 **the guards played cards**: U.S. Congress, "Testimony of Ana María Careaga," 615.

143 **they played Ping-Pong**: Club Atlético was torn down and later excavated by archaeologists who found a Ping-Pong ball in the rubble. Survivors told them that detainees were kept blindfolded, but they could hear Ping-Pong being played somewhere nearby. "The ping-pong ball proved to be a powerful symbol of the whole detention camp system." Andrés Zarankin and Melisa Salerno, "The Engineering of Genocide: An Archaeology of Dictatorship in Argentina," in *Archaeologies of Internment*, eds. Adrian Myers and Gabriel Moshenska (Springer, 2011), 219.

143 **Many of the mothers were very fond**: Fisher, *Mothers of the Disappeared*, 69.

146 **the same blue sweater**: Tina Rosenberg, "The Good Sailor," in *Children of Cain: Violence and the Violent in Latin America* (Penguin Books, 1992), 80.

146 **"He looks like an angel!"**: The family Sister Alice Domon lived with, quoted in Alberto Marquardt, dir., *"Yo, Sor Alice,"* Cine Ojo and Point de Jour, 2001.

146 **He hung on Azucena**: Uki Goñi, *Judas: La Verdadera Historia de Alfredo Astiz, el Infiltrado* (Editorial Sudamericana, 1996), 44, 52; Rosenberg, "Good Sailor," 80.

146 **Gustavo threw himself into the fray**: Goñi, *Judas*, 195–96.

146 **told him it was too dangerous**: Fisher, *Mothers of the Disappeared*, 69.

146 **offered to drive people home**: Goñi, *Judas*, 77; Marquardt, *"Yo, Sor Alice."*

146   **he kissed the Madres goodbye:** Goñi, *Judas*, 11, 86.

146   **Sister Alice asked:** CONADEP, *Nunca Más*, 343.

146   **The *Buenos Aires Herald* announced:** Goñi, *Judas*, 97.

147   **military officials claimed:** CONADEP, *Nunca Más*, 343.

147   **Gustavo Niño returned:** Fisher, *Mothers of the Disappeared*, 69; Rosenberg, "Good Sailor," 81.

147   **Astiz continued his infiltrations:** Goñi, *Judas*, 202–3; Rosenberg, "Good Sailor," 81, 97.

147   **International news agencies circulated:** Goñi, *Judas*, 206; Rosenberg, "Good Sailor," 81–82.

147   **requested his extradition:** Juan E. Méndez, *Truth and Partial Justice in Argentina: An Update*, Human Rights Watch, 1991, 32; Michael A. Meyer, "Liability of Prisoners of War for Offences Committed Prior to Capture: The Astiz Affair," *International and Comparative Law Quarterly* 32, no. 4 (1983).

147   **Dagmar Hagelin:** Méndez, *Truth and Partial Justice*, 31–33; Rosenberg, "Good Sailor," 96–97.

148   **frequently spotted:** Feitlowitz, *Lexicon of Terror*, 256n67, 266, 286; Rosenberg, "Good Sailor," 82, 101.

148   **Astiz's impunity lasted until 2011:** Helen Popper and Karina Grazina, "Life Sentence for Argentine 'Blond Angel of Death,'" Reuters, October 27, 2011.

148   **"I might have made":** Mark Osiel, *Mass Atrocity, Ordinary Evil, and Hannah Arendt: Criminal Consciousness in Argentina's Dirty War* (Yale University Press, 2001), 27.

148   **"People are frightened":** Ibid., 58.

148   **"He's not on the margin":** Ibid.

148   **It was a paperback copy:** Feitlowitz, *Lexicon of Terror*, 308.

148   **"They thought there was only one":** Aída de Suárez, quoted in Arditti, *Searching for Life*, 36.

Chapter 10: Seven Griefs

150   **targeted young people:** Disappeared people between the ages of 21 and 30: 58.52 percent. CONADEP, *Nunca Más*, 285.

150   **The idea that opening graves:** Relevant work on the psychosocial impact of disappearance and exhumation includes Magriet Blaauw and Virpi Lähteenmäki, "Negación y Silencio o Reconocimiento y Revelación de La Información," *Revista Internacional de La Cruz*

Roja no. 848 (2002); Pérez-Sales and Navarro García, *Resistencias Contra el Olvido;* Barbara Preitler, *Grief and Disappearance: Psychosocial Interventions* (SAGE Publications India, 2015); Simon Robins, *Families of the Missing* (Routledge, 2013).

150 **"satisfies the widely held belief":** Renshaw, *Exhuming Loss,* 11.

151 **Who had been found:** For a technical look at sibling identification, see Kornelia Droździok et al., "When DNA Profiling Is Not Enough? A Case of Same-Sex Siblings Identification," *Legal Medicine* 50 (2021); Maeda Kazuho et al., "The Case of 2 Siblings That Identified Not Only by DNA Profiling," *Forensic Science International: Genetics Supplement Series* 5 (2015).

151 **their father had a dream:** A similar story about identification through dreams is documented in Naomi Kinsella and Soren Blau, "Searching for Conflict-Related Missing Persons in Timor-Leste: Technical, Political and Cultural Considerations," *Stability: International Journal of Security and Development* 2, no. 1 (2013).

152 **He peppers his conversation:** As Eva Van Roekel observes, "Many Argentinians have internalized psychoanalysis as a social language" and part of "everyday vocabulary." Eva Van Roekel, *Phenomenal Justice: Violence and Morality in Argentina* (Rutgers University Press, 2020), 75–76.

152 **steeped in psychoanalytic thought:** Jorge Balán, *Cuéntame Tu Vida: Una Biografía Colectiva Del Psicoanálisis Argentino* (Planeta, 1991); Alejandro Dagfal, *Entre París y Buenos Aires: La Invención Del Psicólogo, 1942–1966* (Paidós, 2009); Mariano Ben Plotkin, *Argentina on the Couch: Psychiatry, State, and Society, 1880 to the Present* (University of New Mexico Press, 2003).

152 **According to the World Health Organization:** Argentina has 222 psychologists per 100,000 people; the United States has fewer than 30. World Health Organization, *Atlas of Mental Health Resources in the World 2017,* World Health Organization, 2017. The city of Buenos Aires has more than 1,200 psychologists for every 100,000 inhabitants. Modesto Alonso and Doménica Klinar, *Los Psicólogos en Argentine: Relevamiento Cuantitativo 2014,* VII Congreso Internacional de Investigación y Práctica Profesional en Psicología, Universidad de Buenos Aires, 2014.

152 **Argentine public hospitals:** Juan Eduardo Bonnin, *Discourse and Mental Health: Voice, Inequality and Resistance in Medical Settings* (Routledge, 2018).

152 **Some prisons:** Olivia Goldhill, "Freudian Psychoanalysis Is So Popular in Argentina, Even Prisoners Go Once a Week," *Quartz*, August 20, 2016.

152 **Argentina staunchly clung:** Andrew Lakoff, "The Lacan Ward: Pharmacology and Subjectivity in Buenos Aires," *Social Analysis* 47, no. 2 (2003).

152 **newspaper columns, television talk shows:** Xochitl Marsilli-Vargas, "The Offline and Online Mediatization of Psychoanalysis in Buenos Aires," *Signs and Society* 4, no. 1 (2016).

153 **"The work of mourning":** Darian Leader, *The New Black: Mourning, Melancholia, and Depression* (Graywolf Press, 2009), 172; French psychoanalyst Daniel Lagache echoes this, describing the "aim of mourning" as "killing the dead." Daniel Lagache, *The Works of Daniel Lagache: Selected Writings* (Routledge, 2018), 17.

153 **A complex and controversial figure:** See, for example, Michael Grant, "The Shrink from Hell," in *The Raymond Tallis Reader*, ed. Michael Grant (Palgrave Macmillan, 2000); Stuart Jeffries, "The Great Seducer," *The Spectator*, April 7, 2018.

153 **Lacan has the status:** See, for example, Alejandro Dagfal, "Lacan en la Argentina," *Pagina 12*, September 9, 2021; Germán García, "Lacan, una Pasión Argentina," *Clarín*, September 21, 2006; Jane Russo, "The Lacanian Movement in Argentina and Brazil: The Periphery Becomes the Center," in *The Transnational Unconscious*, eds. Joy Damousi and Mariano Ben Plotkin (Palgrave Macmillan, 2009).

153 **complexity of Lacanian language:** Feitlowitz, *Lexicon of Terror*, 40.

153 **Antigone is the popular saint:** Works on disappearance and exhumation with extended discussion of Antigone include Matt Aho and Mercedes Doretti, dirs., *Following Antigone: Forensic Anthropology and Human Rights Investigations* (Witness, 2002); Jean Bethke Elshtain, "Antigone's Daughters," in *Feminism and Politics*, ed. Anne Phillips (Oxford University Press, 1998); Griselda Gambaro, "Antígona Furiosa," in *Information for Foreigners: Three Plays by Griselda Gambaro*, ed. and trans. Marguerite Feitlowitz (Northwestern University Press, 1992); Nicole Iturriaga, *Exhuming Violent Histories: Forensics, Memory, and Rewriting Spain's Past* (Columbia University Press, 2022); Iosif Kovras, *Grassroots Activism and the Evolution of Transitional Justice: The Families of*

the Disappeared (Cambridge University Press, 2017); Isaias Rojas-Perez, *Mourning Remains: State Atrocity, Exhumations, and Governing the Disappeared in Peru's Postwar Andes* (Stanford University Press, 2017); Paul Sant Cassia, *Bodies of Evidence: Burial, Memory and the Recovery of Missing Persons in Cyprus* (Berghahn Books, 2005); Taylor, *Disappearing Acts.*

154 **"unbearable splendor":** Jacques Lacan and Jacques-Alain Miller, *The Ethics of Psychoanalysis 1959–1960: The Seminar of Jacques Lacan* (Routledge, 2013), 247.

155 **would be to symbolically kill them:** Argentine psychoanalyst María Lucila Pelento echoes this assessment, describing that for a woman named Sonia, whose partner, Raúl, had been disappeared, "accepting that Raúl was dead was equivalent to killing him." María Lucila Pelento, "Mourning for 'Missing' People," in *On Freud's Mourning and Melancholia*, eds. Leticia Glocer de Fiorini, Thierry Bokanowski, and Sergio Lewkowicz (Karnac, 2009), 64.

155 **"After my son and his wife disappeared":** Raquel Marizcurrena, quoted in Arditti, *Searching for Life*, 83.

155 **"They must have done something":** Crenzel, *Memory of the Argentina Disappearances*, 78; Francesca Lessa, *Memory and Transitional Justice in Argentina and Uruguay: Against Impunity* (Springer, 2013), 180.

155 **"anticipatory obedience":** Timothy Snyder, *On Tyranny* (Tim Duggan Books, 2017), 18.

155 **"Most of the power of authoritarianism":** Ibid., 17.

156 SILENCE IS HEALTH: Feitlowitz, *Lexicon of Terror*, 39.

157 **"like the delayed rays":** Roland Barthes, *Camera Lucida: Reflections on Photography* (Macmillan, 1981), 81.

157 **"their strange coolness":** Achille Mbembé, "Necropolitics," *Public Culture* 15, no. 1 (2003): 35.

157 **To recognize a missing person:** This theme is explored in ethnographies of exhumations such as Renshaw, *Exhuming Loss;* Rojas-Perez, *Mourning Remains;* Sant Cassia, *Bodies of Evidence;* Wagner, *To Know Where He Lies.*

158 **One definition of melancholy:** Slavoj Žižek, "Melancholy and the Act," *Critical Inquiry* 26, no. 4 (2000): 662.

159 **"Closure through a traditional funeral":** Louis Bickford et al., *Documenting Truth* (International Center for Transitional Justice, 2009), 29.

159   **From an anthropological point of view:** Antonius C.G.M. Robben, ed., *Death, Mourning, and Burial: A Cross-Cultural Reader* (John Wiley and Sons, 2009).

159   ***Mourning and Melancholia:*** Sigmund Freud, "Mourning and Melancholia," in *The Standard Edition of the Complete Psychological Works of Sigmund Freud*, vol. XIV, *1914–1916*, trans. and ed. James Strachey, with Anna Freud, Alix Strachey, and Alan Tyson (Hogarth Press, 1968).

159   **Psychological theories:** Among others, George A. Bonanno, *The Other Side of Sadness: What the New Science of Bereavement Tells Us About Life After Loss* (Basic Books, 2009); Christine Valentine, *Bereavement Narratives: Continuing Bonds in the Twenty-First Century* (Routledge, 2008).

160   **funeral rites to be culturally universal:** Robben, *Death, Mourning, and Burial*, 9.

160   **"We care for the dead":** Laqueur, *Work of the Dead*, 5.

160   **pathologically "complicated":** Jeanne W. Rothaupt and Kent Becker, "A Literature Review of Western Bereavement Theory: From Decathecting to Continuing Bonds," *The Family Journal* 15, no. 1 (2007); Robert A. Neimeyer et al., *Grief and Bereavement in Contemporary Society: Bridging Research and Practice* (Routledge, 2021).

160   **ordinary German word:** Peter Gay, *Freud: A Life for Our Time* (W. W. Norton, 2006), n465; Thomas W. Laqueur, *Making Sex: Body and Gender from the Greeks to Freud* (Harvard University Press, 1992), 242.

160   **grief cannot come to "normal closure":** Pauline Boss, *Ambiguous Loss* (1999; repr., Harvard University Press, 2009), 10.

160   **"Consider an old woman in Bosnia":** Ibid., 6.

161   **"The absence of the body":** Lucia Corti, "Mourning the Disappeared," *Journal of the Centre for Freudian Analysis and Research* 20 (2010), 12. See also Julia Braun and María Lucila Pelento, "El Proceso de Duelo En Familiares de Desaparecidos: Un Duelo Especial," in *Violencia de Estado y Psicoanálisis*, eds. Janine Puget and René Kaës (Lumen, 2006); Sebastián Luis Piasek, "El Duelo ante la Ausencia del Cuerpo," VII Congreso Internacional de Investigación y Práctica Profesional en Psicología, XXII Jornadas de Investigación XI Encuentro de Investigadores en Psicología del MERCOSUR, Universidad de Buenos Aires, Buenos Aires, 2015.

161 **"face endless melancholia":** Cecilia Taiana, "Mourning the Dead, Mourning the Disappeared: The Enigma of the Absent Presence," *The International Journal of Psychoanalysis* 95, no. 6 (2014): 1104.

161 **"prevents them from mourning":** International Committee of the Red Cross, *The Need to Know: Restoring Links Between Dispersed Family Members,* cited in Victor Toom, "Finding Closure, Continuing Bonds, and Codentification After the 9/11 Attacks," *Medical Anthropology* 37, no. 4 (2018): 268.

161 **"opportunity to mourn":** Interpol, *Disaster Victim Identification Guide,* cited in ibid.

164 **"The disappeared are just that":** Quoted in Finchelstein, *Ideological Origins of the Dirty War,* 133.

165 **"Aparición con vida":** Roberto Amigo Cerisola, "Aparición con Vida: Las Siluetas de Detenidos-Desaparecidos," *Razón y Revolución* 1 (1995); Zoë Crossland, "Violent Spaces: Conflict Over the Reappearance of Argentina's Disappeared," in *Matériel Culture: The Archaeology of Twentieth-Century Conflict,* eds. John Schofield, William Gray Johnson, and Colleen M. Beck (Routledge, 2003); Fisher, *Mothers of the Disappeared,* 128; Rosenblatt, *Digging for the Disappeared,* 93–115.

165 **Not all families of the missing want exhumations:** Alfredo González-Ruibal and Gabriel Moshenska, eds., *Ethics and the Archaeology of Violence* (Springer, 2014), 10.

165 **isn't always widely acknowledged:** Derek Congram and Ariana Fernández, "Uncovering Trauma: The Exhumation and Repatriation of Spanish Civil War Dead," *Anthropology News* 51, no. 3 (2010).

165 **Jewish communities in Poland:** Caroline Sturdy Colls, "Jewish Law, Forensic Investigation, and Archaeology in the Aftermath of the Holocaust," in Brown and Smith, *Routledge Handbook of Religion, Mass Atrocity, and Genocide;* Adam Rosenblatt, "Sacred Graves and Human Rights," in *Human Rights at the Crossroads,* ed. Mark Goodale (Oxford University Press, 2012).

165 **"We would choose to leave Lorca":** Quoted in Rosenblatt, *Digging for the Disappeared,* 68.

165 **at an early exhumation:** Salama, *Tumbas Anónimas.*

166 **"It was hard to see":** Quoted in Guerriero, "El Rastro en los Huesos."

166 **"Many want the wound to dry":** Quoted in Antonius C.G.M. Rob-

ben, "How Traumatized Societies Remember: The Aftermath of Argentina's Dirty War," *Cultural Critique* 59, no. 1 (2005): 144.

166   **political melancholia:** For more on the politics of mourning, see David L. Eng and David Kazanjian, eds., *Loss: The Politics of Mourning* (University of California Press, 2003); Everett Yuehong Zhang, "Mourning," in *A Companion to Moral Anthropology*, ed. Didier Fassin (John Wiley and Sons, 2015); Lochlann Jain, "Living in Prognosis: Toward an Elegiac Politics," *Representations* 98, no. 1 (2007); Judith Butler, *Precarious Life: The Powers of Mourning and Violence* (Verso Books, 2004).

166   **the Madres split:** Fernando J. Bosco, "Human Rights Politics and Scaled Performances of Memory: Conflicts Among the Madres de Plaza de Mayo in Argentina," *Social and Cultural Geography* 5, no. 3 (2004).

166   **"Grieving breaks us apart":** Cristina Rivera Garza,. *Grieving: Dispatches from a Wounded Country* (Feminist Press, 2020), 16.

166   **Believing his father to be among the dead:** María Laura Martín Chiappe, "Micropolíticas del Entierro Digno: Exhumaciones Contemporáneas de Víctimas del Franquismo y Culturas Memoriales Transnacionales en el Valle del Tiéta" (PhD diss., Universidad Autónoma de Madrid, 2020), 110. For more on family conflicts during exhumations in Spain, see Rachel Carmen Ceasar, "Kinship Across Conflict: Family Blood, Political Bones, and Exhumation in Contemporary Spain," *Social Dynamics* 42, no. 2 (2016).

167   **"This is a thing that the whole world":** Laura Panizo, "Among Bodies: Reflections on Ethnographic Work and the Repercussions of Exhumations and Identifications of the Disappeared of the Last Military Dictatorship in Argentina," *Human Remains and Violence: An Interdisciplinary Journal* 2, no. 2 (2016): 30.

167   **"That ritual, that burial, was a denunciation":** Ibid.

167   **the angel of history:** Walter Benjamin, "On the Concept of History," in *Illuminations: Essays and Reflections* (Houghton Mifflin Harcourt, 2019).

167   **Reflecting on his original views:** Sigmund Freud, *The Ego and the Id* (W. W. Norton, 1989), 23.

167   **Rather than see melancholy:** Tammy Clewell, "Mourning Beyond Melancholia: Freud's Psychoanalysis of Loss," *Journal of the American Psychoanalytic Association* 52, no. 1 (2004).

167   ***"We are our memory":*** Jorge Luis Borges, "Cambridge," in *Selected Poems*, ed. Alexander Coleman (Penguin Books, 1999).

168 **"Sunday Child":** Jacqueline Rose, "To Die One's Own Death," *London Review of Books,* November 19, 2020.

168 **"We know that the acute sorrow":** Sigmund Freud to Ludwig Binswanger, April 11, 1929, in *Letters of Sigmund Freud,* ed. Ernst L. Freud (Dover, 1992).

168 **beloved is not "replaced":** Salman Akhtar, "Bereavement: The Spectrum of Emotional Reactions," in *Bereavement: Personal Experiences and Clinical Reflections,* eds. Salman Akhtar and Gurmeet S. Kanwal (Routledge, 2018), 5.

168 **call closure "a myth":** Pauline Boss, "Ambiguous Loss Research, Theory, and Practice: Reflections After 9/11," *Journal of Marriage and Family* 66, no. 3 (2004): 560; Pauline Boss, *The Myth of Closure: Ambiguous Loss in a Time of Pandemic and Change* (W. W. Norton, 2021).

168 **most found resolution:** Boss, "Ambiguous Loss Research"; Pauline Boss, "Ambiguous Loss: Working with Families of the Missing," *Family Process* 41, no. 1 (2002).

168 **Recent psychological research:** Rothaupt and Becker, "A Literature Review of Western Bereavement Theory"; Neimeyer et al., *Grief and Bereavement.*

169 **continues to be informed:** Toom, "Finding Closure"; Laura Panizo, "Cuerpos Desaparecidos: La Ubicación Ritual de la Muerte Desatendida," in *Etnografías de la Muerte,* ed. Cecilia Hidalgo (CLASCO, 2011); Manon Bourguignon, Alice Dermitzel, and Muriel Katz, "Grief Among Relatives of Disappeared Persons in the Context of State Violence: An Impossible Process?," *Torture Journal* 31, no. 2 (2021).

Chapter 11: Southern Cross

170 **the question "Which Catholicism?":** This question is explored at length in Morello, *Catholic Church and Argentina's Dirty War.*

170 **relationship of "symbiosis":** Fortunato Mallimaci and Juan Cruz Esquivel, "The Triad of State, Religious Institutions and Civil Society in Modern Argentina," *Amerika: Mémoires, Identités, Territoires* 8 (2013): para. 39.

171 **90 percent Catholic:** Morello, *Catholic Church and Argentina's Dirty War,* 1.

171 **"the cross and the sword":** Finchelstein, *Ideological Origins of the Dirty War,* 40.

171   **state even paid the salaries:** Ibid., 160.

171   **"Third World Priest Movement":** José Pablo Martín, "El Movimiento de Sacerdotes para el Tercer Mundo: Un Debate Argentino en Nuevo Mundo," *Revista de Teología Latinoamericana* (1992); Fortunato Mallimaci, "Le Catholicisme Argentin de Bergoglio et le Pontificat de François: Une Première Approximation Depuis l'Argentine," *Problèmes d'Amérique Latine* 2 (2018).

171   **church openly defied:** Emelio Betances, *The Catholic Church and Power Politics in Latin America: The Dominican Case in Comparative Perspective* (Rowman and Littlefield, 2007).

171   **"decisive overwhelming support":** Finchelstein, *Ideological Origins of the Dirty War,* 9.

171   **"Will Christ not wish":** Quoted in Mignone, "Catholic Church, Human Rights," 356.

172   **clergy were close to the junta:** Feitlowitz, *Lexicon of Terror,* 256; Finchelstein, *Ideological Origins of the Dirty War,* 159; Mignone, "Catholic Church, Human Rights," 355.

172   **"excellent, very cordial":** Quoted in Ricardo Angoso García, "Entrevista a Jorge Rafael Videla: 'En Argentina no Hay Justicia, Sino Venganza, que es Otra Cosa, Bien Distinta,'" *Cambio 16,* February 20, 2012.

172   **"they advised us":** Quoted in "Videla afirma que la Iglesia conocía las desapariciones," *Diario Sur,* July 22, 2012.

172   **The work is part:** Juan Ignacio Provéndola, "Las Mil y Una Obras de Adolfo Pérez Esquivel," *Pagina 12,* November 26, 2019.

173   **His sermons:** Michael Dodson, "Priests and Peronism: Radical Clergy and Argentine Politics," *Latin American Perspectives* 1, no. 3 (1974): 68; see also Morello, *Catholic Church and Argentina's Dirty War,* 26, 61–62.

173   **he was assassinated:** Finchelstein, *Ideological Origins of the Dirty War,* 117.

173   **Bishop Enrique Ángel Angelelli Carletti:** CONADEP, *Nunca Más,* 350–52; Morello, *Catholic Church and Argentina's Dirty War,* 32–33.

173   **In the city of Córdoba:** Morello, *Catholic Church and Argentina's Dirty War;* U.S. Congress, *Human Rights in Argentina: Hearings Before the Subcommittee on International Organizations of the Committee on International Relations, House of Representatives, Ninety-fourth Congress, Second Session, September 28 and 29, 1976* (U.S. Government Printing Office, 1976), 2–7.

174 **General Videla's son:** Seoane and Muleiro, *El Dictador,* 334; "Videla y las Monjas Francesas, un Vínculo entre la Caridad y la Impiedad," *Clarín,* September 4, 2005.

174 **Alice lived in Villa 20:** Marquardt, *"Yo, Sor Alice"*; Frédéric Santangelo, *Se Taire Serait Lâche* (Editions du Panthéon, 2021), 24; Diana Beatriz Viñoles, "Espacio-tiempo en la Existencia de Alice Domon (1937–1977): Una Biografía Filosófica," *Sociedad y Religión* 24, no. 42 (2014); Diana Beatriz Viñoles, *Lettres d'Alice Domon, une Disparue d'Argentine* (Karthala, 2016).

174 **"The persecution grows worse":** Letter dated September 19, 1976, quoted in Marquardt, *"Yo, Sor Alice."*

174 **"It is interesting that suffering":** Letter dated November 8, 1977, quoted in Marquardt, *"Yo, Sor Alice"* and Santangelo, *Se Taire Serait Lâche,* 141–42.

175 **"an angel with black wings":** Alejandro Dausá, quoted in Morello, *Catholic Church and Argentina's Dirty War,* 121.

175 **"You are not a guerrilla":** Quoted in Mignone, "Catholic Church, Human Rights," 369.

175 **"you unite the poor":** Ibid.

175 **The false priest lectured:** Morello, *Catholic Church and Argentina's Dirty War,* 121–22.

175 **"The Silence of the Bishops":** Cox, *Dirty Secrets, Dirty War,* 88; Goñi, *Judas,* 62–63.

175 **The group's documentation:** Crenzel, *Memory of the Argentina Disappearances,* 39–43; Robben, *Political Violence and Trauma,* 323; Elizabeth Jelin, "The Politics of Memory: The Human Rights Movement and the Construction of Democracy in Argentina," *Latin American Perspectives* 21, no. 2 (1994).

175 **executed at Saint Patrick's Church:** Cox, *Dirty Secrets, Dirty War,* 88–89; U.S. Congress, *Human Rights in Argentina,* 29.

175 **priests at Iglesia Santa Cruz heard:** Goñi, *Judas,* 62.

176 **"These lefties died":** Morello, *Catholic Church and Argentina's Dirty War,* 81–82.

176 **"Subversive elements":** "Preocupación Tras el Asesinato de Cinco Religiosos en Buenos Aires," *El País,* July 6, 1976.

176 **"El Cura":** Feitlowitz, *Lexicon of Terror,* 27.

176 **"Come, my child":** Ibid., 69.

176 **real priests visited:** Finchelstein, *Ideological Origins of the Dirty War,* 130–32.

176 **Christian Federico Von Wernich:** Margarita K. O'Donnell, "New

Dirty War Judgments in Argentina: National Courts and Domestic Prosecutions of International Human Rights Violations," *New York University Law Review* 84 (2009); Sam Ferguson, "Priest Convicted in Argentine 'Dirty War' Tribunal," *Yale Law School Report,* October 10, 2007.

176 **"God wants to know":** Jonathan Watts and Uki Goñi, "New Pope's Role During Argentina's Military Era Disputed," *The Guardian,* March 15, 2013.

176 **"The worst torture I suffered":** Testimony of Rúben Schell, quoted in "'La Peor Tortura fue la Moral,' Dijo un Testigo," *La Nación,* August 6, 2007.

176 **washing blood off his hands:** Patrick J. McDonnell, "The Priest Who Helped in Murders, Torture," *SFGATE,* October 28, 2007.

176 **"Father Von Wernich saw":** CONADEP, *Nunca Más,* 249.

177 **"When we had doubts":** Mignone, *Witness to the Truth,* 11.

177 **Priests and chaplains reassured torturers:** Osiel, *Mass Atrocity, Ordinary Evil, and Hannah Arendt,* 104–48.

177 **church did not excommunicate:** Feitlowitz, *Lexicon of Terror,* 322.

177 **participated in a conspiracy of silence:** Finchelstein, *Ideological Origins of the Dirty War,* 160.

177 **accuse him of active collaboration:** Horacio Verbitsky, *El Silencio: De Paulo VI a Bergoglio: Las Relaciones Secretas de la Iglesia con la ESMA* (Editorial Sudamericana, 2005).

177 **claim he acted with quiet resistance:** "Pérez Esquivel: 'El Papa No Tenía Vínculos Con La Dictadura,'" BBC Mundo, March 14, 2013; Vladimir Hernandez, "Argentina 'Dirty War' Accusations Haunt Pope Francis," BBC Mundo, March 15, 2013.

177 **torture of two priests:** María Soledad Catoggio, "Argentine Catholicism During the Last Military Dictatorship: Unresolved Tensions and Tragic Outcomes," *Journal of Latin American Cultural Studies* 22, no. 2 (2013).

177 **"I realized I was":** CONADEP, *Nunca Más,* 345.

178 **In a second case:** Watts and Goñi, "New Pope's Role"; Arditti, *Searching for Life,* 57.

178 **"knew what was happening":** Daniel Politi, "Priest Details Arrest During Argentine Dirty War but Doesn't Comment on Pope Francis' Role," McClatchy Washington Bureau, March 15, 2013.

178 **"Perhaps he didn't have":** Watts and Goñi, "New Pope's Role."

178 **"Orlando Yorio and I":** William Neuman, "'Dirty War' Victim Rejects Pope's Connection to Kidnapping," *The New York Times*, March 22, 2013; Jonathan Watts, "Pope Francis Did Not Denounce Me to Argentinian Junta, Says Priest," *The Guardian*, March 21, 2013.

178 **"I am reconciled":** "Erklärung von Pater Franz Jalics SJ," *Jesuiten IHS*, May 6, 2013.

179 **"When I hear him speak":** Quoted in Uki Goñi, "Opinion: The Peronist Roots of Pope Francis' Politics," *The New York Times*, August 12, 2015.

179 **"She's the person":** Ailín Bullentini, "La Madre de Ustedes Me Enseñó a Pensar," *Pagina 12*, July 12, 2015.

181 **"bless" means "to mark":** The OED says, "*Original meaning* (probably), To make 'sacred' or 'holy' with blood." Oxford English Dictionary, *OED Online* (Oxford University Press, March 2022).

181 **bodies washed up:** CONADEP, *Nunca Más*, 223; Equipo Argentino de Antropología Forense, *Annual Report 2006* (EAAF, 2006), 34.

181 **Declassified documents:** "US Declassified Documents: Argentine Junta Security Forces Killed, Disappeared Activists, Mothers and Nuns," National Security Archives, December 8, 2002.

181 **exhumed a section of the cemetery:** EAAF, *Annual Report 2006*, 33–38.

181 **tomb twenty-three:** Celesia, *La Muerte es el Olvido*, 154.

182 **"These mothers, tireless fighters":** "Emotivo Homenaje a Azucena Villaflor y a Otras dos Madres de Plaza de Mayo," *Clarín*, July 25, 2005; "Declaran Sitio Histórico a La Iglesia de La Santa Cruz," *Parque Chas Web*, November 9, 2007.

182 **"A little while ago we received news":** U.S. Congress, "Testimony of Ana María Careaga," 616.

Chapter 12: Odysseus

185 *"No, you don't understand":* Verbitsky, *Confessions of an Argentine Dirty Warrior*, 2.

185 **given a "vaccination":** Ibid., 21–22.

185 **"Something to do with the Hippocratic":** Ibid., 52.

185 **"kind of communion":** Ibid., 23.

185 **"Christian death":** Ibid., 30.

185 **When his confession went public:** For an example of coverage in

the United States, see Calvin Sims, "Argentine Tells of Dumping 'Dirty War' Captives into Sea," *The New York Times,* March 13, 1995.

186 **Argentina had drifted into denialism:** See Robben, *Argentina Betrayed;* Barbara Sutton and Kari Marie Norgaard, "Cultures of Denial: Avoiding Knowledge of State Violations of Human Rights in Argentina and the United States," *Sociological Forum* 28, no. 3 (2013).

186 **Scilingo's admission prompted a confrontation:** Including other confessions, known as the "Scilingo Effect." Feitlowitz, *Lexicon of Terror,* 164.

186 **patterns of skeletal trauma:** Equipo Argentino de Antropología Forense, *Annual Report 2005* (EAAF, 2005), 48; Antonius C.G.M. Robben and Francisco J. Ferrándiz, "The Transitional Lives of Crimes Against Humanity Forensic Evidence Under Changing Political Circumstances," in *Bodies as Evidence: Security, Knowledge, and Power,* eds. Mark Maguire, Ursula Rao, and Nils Zurawski (Duke University Press, 2018), 122.

186 **In falls, trauma is determined:** In this section, I draw from Suzanne M. Abel and Scott Ramsey, "Patterns of Skeletal Trauma in Suicidal Bridge Jumpers: A Retrospective Study from the Southeastern United States," *Forensic Science International* 231, nos. 1–3 (2013); Samantha K. Rowbotham et al., "An Assessment of the Skeletal Fracture Patterns Resulting from Fatal High (>3 m) Free Falls," *Journal of Forensic Sciences* 64, no. 1 (2019).

187 **"Physical pain does not simply resist":** Elaine Scarry, *The Body in Pain: The Making and Unmaking of the World* (Oxford University Press, 1987), 4.

187 **Miriam Lewin began investigating:** Giancarlo Ceraudo and Miriam Lewin, *Destino Final* (Shilt Publishing, 2017); Miriam Lewin, *Skyvan: Aviones, Pilotos y Archivos Secretos* (Penguin Random House Grupo Editorial Argentina, 2017).

188 **"a golden discovery":** Quoted in "'Death Flights' Trial Opens in Argentina," Reuters, November 28, 2012.

188 **The flight is believed:** Natalia Chientaroli, "Cadena Perpetua para los Responsables de los 'Vuelos de la Muerte' de la Dictadura Argentina," *El Diario,* November 30, 2017; Uki Goñi, "Argentina 'Death Flight' Pilots Sentenced for Deaths Including Pope's Friend," *The Guardian,* November 29, 2017.

188 **the trial of pilots:** A third pilot, Enrique José de Saint George, died during the trial.

188 **he was arrested on charges:** Verbitsky, *Confessions of an Argentine Dirty Warrior*, 180–81.

188 **Spain recognizes no national:** Joseph Rikhof, *A Theory of Punishable Participation in Universal Crimes* (Torkel Opsahl, 2018).

188 **1,084-year prison sentence:** "Un Tribunal Español Condenó a Scilingo a 1.084 Años de Prisión," *Clarín*, July 5, 2007.

189 **Among the most important:** "Megacausa ESMA: El Jucio," *Especiales, Centro de Estudios Legales y Sociales CELS* (2017). For an in-depth consideration of the meaning of trials, see Van Roekel, *Phenomenal Justice.*

190 **telling of the Trojan War:** Albert Bates Lord, *The Singer of Tales* (Harvard University Press, 1960).

191 **No one now knows the melodies:** Scholars including Georg Danek of the University of Vienna and Stefan Hagel of the Austrian Academy of Sciences have tried to re-create the songs. "Hear What Homer's *Odyssey* Sounded Like When Sung in the Original Ancient Greek," *Open Culture*, October 21, 2016.

Chapter 13: The Guarumo Tree

192 **many mass graves were in wells:** In Latin America, "empty water wells" are common sites of clandestine graves. Fondebrider, "Forensic Anthropology and the Investigation of Political Violence," 43.

192 **In Spain, the bodies:** Francisco Etxeberria et al., "Contemporary Exhumations in Spain: Recovering the Missing from the Spanish Civil War," in *Forensic Archaeology: A Global Perspective*, eds. W. J. Mike Groen, Nicholas Marquez-Grant, and Rob Janaway (John Wiley and Sons, 2015), 497; Francisco Ferrándiz, "Mass Graves, Landscapes of Terror," in Ferrándiz and Robben, *Necropolitics*, 110.

192 **war in Croatia:** Mario Šlaus et al., "Identification and Analysis of Human Remains Recovered from Wells from the 1991 War in Croatia," *Forensic Science International* 171, no. 1 (2007).

192 **Forensic teams in Cyprus:** Deren Ceker and William D. Stevens, "Recovery of Missing Persons in Cyprus: Heavy Equipment Methods and Techniques for Complex Well Excavations," *Journal of Forensic Sciences* 60, no. 6 (2015).

192 **"easy and obvious choice":** Ibid., 1529.

192 **A guarumo tree:** Aura Elena Farfán, interview, *This American Life,* "What Happened at Dos Erres," episode 465, May 25, 2012; Louisa Reynolds, *The Long Road to Justice: Survivors of the Dos Erres Massacre Tell Their Story* (Plaza Publica, 2013), 30.

193 **Invited by Guatemalan human rights groups:** CLACSO, *Ciencia por la Verdad,* 57.

193 **activist Aura Elena Farfán:** Reynolds, *Long Road to Justice,* 35–36; Farfán interview, *This American Life.*

193 **The team began to dig:** In telling the story of the exhumation of Dos Erres, my primary sources are interviews with Fredy Peccerelli and Luis Fondebrider, and the following texts: Amnesty International, "Victims of 1982 Army Massacre at Las Dos Erres Exhumed," November 1, 1995; "Massacre at Las Dos Erres," CEH, *Memory of Silence,* 50–52; Equipo Argentino de Antropología Forense, *Annual Report,* "Guatemala" (1998 and 1999); Inter-American Court of Human Rights, *Case of the "Las Dos Erres" Massacre v. Guatemala,* Judgment of November 24, 2009; Darío Olmo, "Crimes Against Humanity," in *Forensic Anthropology and Medicine,* eds. Aurore Schmitt, Eugénia Cunha, and João Pinheiro (Humana Press, 2006).

193 **Their actual transgression:** Simone Remijnse, *Memories of Violence: Civil Patrols and the Legacy of Conflict in Joyabaj, Guatemala* (Purdue University Press, 2002); CEH, *Memory of Silence,* 117–23; Jean-Marie Simon, *Civil Patrols in Guatemala,* Americas Watch Report, August 1986; Inter-American Court of Human Rights, *Case of the "Las Dos Erres" Massacre.*

194 **U.S. President Ronald Reagan:** "Remarks in San Pedro Sula, Honduras, Following a Meeting with President Jose Efrain Rios Montt of Guatemala," December 4, 1982, *The American Presidency Project,* University of California, Santa Barbara; "Guatemala Is Said to Pledge Elimination of 'Death Squads,'" *The New York Times,* December 7, 1982.

194 **depth of about thirteen feet:** Olmo, "Crimes Against Humanity," 425; Reynolds, *Long Road to Justice,* 36–37; Farfán interview, *This American Life.*

194 **Dos Erres was a new settlement:** Reynolds, *Long Road to Justice;* Sebastian Rotella, "Finding Oscar: Massacre, Memory and Justice in Guatemala," *ProPublica,* May 25, 2012.

194 **"All of the minors":** CEH, *Memory of Silence,* 50.

195 **"they found a hand sticking out":** Ibid., 52.

195 **At twenty-six feet:** Olmo, "Crimes Against Humanity," 425.

195 **The plans they had made:** CLASCO, *Ciencia por la Verdad*, 58.

196 **"Recovery of victims' remains":** Mario Šlaus et al., "Contribution of Forensic Anthropology to Identification Process in Croatia: Examples of Victims Recovered in Wells," *Croatian Medical Journal* 48, no. 4 (2007): 504–5.

196 **"all well excavations":** Ceker and Stevens, "Recovery of Missing Persons in Cyprus," 1532.

196 **"under the supervision":** Ibid.

196 **At Pozo de Vargas:** Ataliva, Gerónimo, and Zurita, *Arqueología Forense y Procesos de Memorias.*

196 **To work safely:** Ceker and Stevens, "Recovery of Missing Persons in Cyprus," 1529–33.

196 **"physical and mental strength":** Ibid., 1532.

196 **Working deep in the well:** Reynolds, *Long Road to Justice*, 37.

197 **"like eggshells":** Ibid.

197 **harassed and threatened:** Amnesty International, "Victims of 1982 Army Massacre."

197 **The prosecutor in charge:** CEH, *Memory of Silence*, 52.

197 **"fractures compatible with lesions":** Olmo, "Crimes Against Humanity," 427.

197 **peri- and postmortem fractures:** Ibid., 428.

197 **women and children:** Ibid., 427.

197 **At the very bottom:** Network in Solidarity with the People of Guatemala, "Las Dos Erres Massacre Case Advances with a New Trial," NISGUA blog, December 12, 2016.

197 **"The massacre of Dos Erres marked":** Ibid.

198 **Rubén Amílcar Farfán:** Gabriela Grijalva Menéndez, "¿Dónde Está Rubén Amílcar Farfán? Aproximación a su Caso Bajo la Luz del Archivo de la Policía de Guatemala," *Trinchera Histórica: Centro de Investigaciones Sobre América Latina y el Caribe*, Universidad Nacional Autónoma de México, June 3, 2021.

198 **at the city morgue:** Henderson, "Seeking Justice in Guatemala," 53, 62; Reynolds, *Long Road to Justice*, 33–34.

198 **Rubén's photo:** Menéndez, "¿Dónde Está Rubén Amílcar Farfán?"

198 **"Peace will not come to Guatemala":** Quoted in Equipo Argentino de Antropología Forense, *Annual Report 1999* (EAAF, 1999), 45.

198 **Clyde Snow began investigating:** Peccerelli and Henderson, "Forensics and Maya Ceremonies," 309.

198 **The Guatemalan team:** Until 1997 the team was called Equipo de Antropología Forense de Guatemala (EAFG). For simplicity I use FAFG throughout the text.

199 **Plan de Sánchez:** Inter-American Court of Human Rights, *Case of Plan de Sánchez Massacre v. Guatemala,* Judgment of April 29, 2004, 14.

199 **"The thing that most people":** Sanford, *Buried Secrets,* 33.

199 **"If anyone wanted to commit murder":** Quoted in Americas Watch Committee and Physicians for Human Rights, "Guatemala: Getting Away with Murder."

200 **read the book:** Rigoberta Menchú, *I, Rigoberta Menchú: An Indian Woman in Guatemala* (Verso Books, 2010). In 1998, Rigoberta Menchú's testimonio was at the center of a controversy when anthropologist David Stoll accused her of factual inaccuracies. David Stoll, *Rigoberta Menchú and the Story of All Poor Guatemalans* (Routledge, 2018). Greg Grandin writes, "More than a decade after the scandal, what is notable about *I, Rigoberta Menchú* is not its exaggerations but its realism." Greg Grandin, *Who Is Rigoberta Menchú?* (Verso Books, 2011), 19. For more on the controversy, see Arturo Arias, ed., *The Rigoberta Menchú Controversy* (University of Minnesota Press, 2001); John Beverley, "Testimonio, Subalternity, and Narrative Authority," in *A Companion to Latin American Literature and Culture,* ed. Sara Castro-Klaren (John Wiley and Sons, 2022); Victoria Sanford, "Between Rigoberta Menchú and La Violencia: Deconstructing David Stoll's History of Guatemala," *Latin American Perspectives* 26, no. 6 (1999).

202 **pioneered methods of forensic statistics:** Clyde Snow and Maria Julia Bihurriet, "An Epidemiology of Homicide: Ningún Nombre Burials in the Province of Buenos Aires from 1970 to 1984," in *Human Rights and Statistics: Getting the Record Straight,* eds. Thomas B. Jabine and Richard Pierre Claude (University of Pennsylvania Press, 2016).

202 **in Guatemala, Clyde discovered:** Snow et al., "Hidden in Plain Sight."

203 **"Regrettably, some of the remains":** Equipo Argentino de Antropología Forense, *Annual Report 2006,* 19.

204 **Silvana Turner from the Argentine team:** Jo-Marie Burt and Paulo Estrada, "Trial Against Ex Kaibil in Massacre of 200 Villagers Nears Conclusion," *International Justice Monitor,* November 20, 2018.

204 **Forty percent of the bodies recovered:** Ibid.

204 **Ramiro Osorio Cristales:** For the incredible story of two boys who survived the Dos Erres massacre, see Rotella, "Finding Oscar"; Farfán interview, *This American Life.* The story was also made into a 2016 feature-length documentary, *Finding Oscar,* directed by Ryan Suffern, with Steven Spielberg as executive producer.

204 **neighbors visited the destroyed settlement:** Reynolds, *Long Road to Justice,* 29–30.

205 **María Esperanza Arreaga ventured:** Ibid.

205 **Saúl Arévalo searched:** Ibid.

205 **Known for its fast growth:** Rafael Ocampo, ed., *Domesticación de Plantas Medicinales en Centroamerica* (CATIE, 1994); James A. Duke, Mary Jo Bogenschutz-Godwin, and Andrea R. Ottesen, eds., *Duke's Handbook of Medicinal Plants of Latin America* (CRC Press, 2008).

205 **Fredy received a note:** Amnesty International, "Urgent Action: Experts Who Testified in Trial Threatened," Index AMR 34/008/2011), August 11, 2011.

205 **"The end of the armed conflict":** Quoted in Diane M. Nelson, *Who Counts? The Mathematics of Death and Life After Genocide* (Duke University Press, 2015), 116.

205 **The largest massacre:** "La Matanza de 27 Campesinos Conmociona a Guatemala," *El País,* May 16, 2011.

206 **no involvement in narcotrafficking:** Assessment of the Guatemalan Ministry of Interior Carlos Menocal quoted in "Guatemala Responsabiliza a Zetas de Masacre," *El Universal,* May 16, 2011; also quoted in Renata Avila, "Guatemala: Brutalidad e Impunidad: Más de 28 Decapitados en Petén," *Global Voices,* May 18, 2011.

206 **Among the Zetas:** George W. Grayson, "The Evolution of Los Zetas in Mexico and Central America: Sadism as an Instrument of Cartel Warfare," U.S. Army War College, Strategic Studies Institute, April 2014; Tim Padgett, "Guatemala's Kaibiles: A Notorious Commando Unit Wrapped Up in Central America's Drug War," *Time,* July 14, 2011.

206 **Kaibiles were named:** Randal C. Archibold, "Guatemala Shooting Raises Concerns About Military's Expanded Role," *The New York Times,* October 20, 2012; Kate Doyle, "The Pursuit of Justice in Guatemala," *National Security Archive Electronic Briefing Book* No. 373, March 23, 2012.

206 **corridor for trafficking:** Steven Dudley, "The Zetas in Guate-

mala," *InSight, Organized Crime in the Americas,* September 8, 2011; Óscar Martínez, "The Lost Border in the Jungle," *El País English Edition,* October 11, 2019.

206 **"commit crimes and acts of terror":** Gladys Tzul Tzul, "The Continuity of Exploitation in Central America," *NACLA Report on the Americas* 48, no. 2 (2016): 139.

206 **parallels with Dos Erres:** Padgett, "Guatemala's Kaibiles"; Reynolds, *Long Road to Justice,* 72.

206 **"The violence of today":** Tzul Tzul, "Continuity of Exploitation," 39.

207 **"We can't separate":** Quoted in International Crisis Group, "Guatemala: Drug Trafficking and Violence," *Latin America Report* 39, October 11, 2011.

207 **"the bodies still wearing":** Óscar Martínez, *A History of Violence: Living and Dying in Central America* (Verso Books, 2016), 114.

Chapter 14: The Well

209 **In archaeological terms:** For archaeological details of the site, see Ataliva et al., "Arqueología Forense Desde las Profundidades."

210 **physical expressions of psychological suffering:** Some examples of this body of literature: Laurence J. Kirmayer, "The Body's Insistence on Meaning: Metaphor as Presentation and Representation in Illness Experience," *Medical Anthropology Quarterly* 6, no. 4 (1992); Arthur Kleinman, *The Illness Narratives: Suffering, Healing, and the Human Condition* (Basic Books, 1998); Nancy Scheper-Hughes and Margaret Lock, "The Mindful Body: A Prolegomenon to Future Work in Medical Anthropology," *Medical Anthropology Quarterly* 1, no. 1 (1987); Shigehisa Kuriyama, *The Expressiveness of the Body and the Divergence of Greek and Chinese Medicine* (Zone Books, 1999); Mark Nichter, "Idioms of Distress Revisited," *Culture, Medicine, and Psychiatry* 34, no. 2 (2010).

211 **"We all have other ambitions":** Stephen G. Michaud, "Identifying Argentina's Disappeared," *The New York Times,* December 27, 1987.

212 **In many sacred traditions:** Alan Dundes, "The Folklore of Wishing Wells," *American Imago* 19, no. 1 (1962); Gary R. Varner, *Sacred Wells: A Study in the History, Meaning, and Mythology of Holy Wells and Waters* (Algora Publishing, 2009).

213 **fountains of Rome:** "Trevi Coins to Fund Food for Poor," BBC News, November 27, 2006.

213   **I grew up believing:** David W. Hughes, "On Seeing Stars Especially Up Chimneys," *Quarterly Journal of the Royal Astronomical Society* 24 (1983).

213   **underground belonged to deities:** Ellie Mackin Roberts, *Underworld Gods in Ancient Greek Religion: Death and Reciprocity* (Routledge, 2020).

213   **"ecstatic illumination":** Yulia Ustinova, *Caves and the Ancient Greek Mind: Descending Underground in the Search for Ultimate Truth* (Oxford University Press, 2009), 52.

213   **sensory deprivation:** Oliver J. Mason and Francesca Brady, "The Psychotomimetic Effects of Short-Term Sensory Deprivation," *The Journal of Nervous and Mental Disease* 197, no. 10 (2009).

213   **monks meditate:** Alan Klima, *The Funeral Casino: Buddhist Meditation, State Terrorism, and Public Images in Thailand* (Princeton University Press, 1996); Todd LeRoy Perreira, "'Die Before You Die': Death Meditation as Spiritual Technology of the Self in Islam and Buddhism," *The Muslim World* 100, nos. 2–3 (2010).

213   **philosopher and mystic al-Ghazali:** Abdulgafar O. Fahm, "Brief Analysis of the Meditation on Death in Sufism: With Reference to Al-Ghazālī and Rūmī," *International Journal of Religion and Spirituality in Society* 4, no. 3 (2014); Nilou Davoudi, "Remember Death: An Examination of Death, Mourning, and Death Anxiety Within Islam," *Open Theology* 8, no. 1 (2022); Abu Hamid Al-Ghazali, "The Remembrance of Death and the Afterlife," trans. T. J. Winter (Islamic Texts Society, 1989).

213   **"To philosophize":** Simon Critchley, "To Philosophize Is to Learn How to Die," *The New York Times,* April 11, 2020; Arthur C. Brooks, "To Be Happier, Start Thinking More About Your Death," *The New York Times,* January 9, 2016.

214   **"Can an anthropology of dying":** Robert Desjarlais, *Subject to Death: Life and Loss in a Buddhist World* (University of Chicago Press, 2021), 19.

216   **reference samples:** Thomas J. Parsons et al., "Large Scale DNA Identification: The ICMP Experience." *Forensic Science International: Genetics* 38 (2019): 242 (table 4).

216   **tons of debris:** Toom, "Whose Body Is It?," 7.

216   **hallmarks of lamentation is its excess:** Veena Das, considering the violence of the Partition of India in 1947, writes of the "excess of speech in the mourning laments and the theatrical infliction of harm on the body" enacted by women. Das, *Life and Words,* 50.

217 **"very act of cordoning off":** Zoë Crossland, "The Archaeology of Contemporary Conflict," in *The Oxford Handbook of the Archaeology of Ritual and Religion*, ed. Timothy Insoll (Oxford University Press, 2011), 287. Exhumations are, in Crossland's words, "sense-making acts." Ibid.

218 **The word "posthumous":** The Oxford English Dictionary explains that in classical Latin, *postumus* means "child born after the father's death," and "posthumous" came to be associated in folk-etymology with *humus*, earth, or *humāre*, to bury. *OED Online* (Oxford University Press, March 2022).

218 **Some scholars even trace a connection:** Robert Pogue Harrison, *The Dominion of the Dead* (University of Chicago Press, 2003), xi.

218 **"To be human is to bury":** Ibid.

218 **"She was lying on her left side":** Koff, *Bone Woman*, 45–47.

219 **"As I troweled down":** Joyce, "Grave Responsibilities," 171.

219 **In most cultures, funeral rituals:** Maurice Bloch and Jonathan Parry, eds., *Death and the Regeneration of Life* (Cambridge University Press, 1982); Peter Metcalf and Richard Huntington, *Celebrations of Death: The Anthropology of Mortuary Ritual* (Cambridge University Press, 1991); Robben, *Death, Mourning, and Burial*.

220 **"part of the production of the sacred":** Crossland, "Archaeology of Contemporary Conflict," 297.

220 **funerals as rites of passage:** Hertz's work predates Arnold van Gennep, *The Rites of Passage* (University of Chicago Press, 1961). See Douglas J. Davies, "Robert Hertz: The Social Triumph Over Death," *Mortality* 5, no. 1 (2000): 99. Hertz's theories of funeral rituals have been applied to exhumations in the works of István Rév, "Parallel Autopsies," *Representations* 49 (1995), and Katherine Verdery, *The Political Lives of Dead Bodies: Reburial and Post-socialist Change* (Columbia University Press, 1999).

220 **"Death is not completed":** Robert Hertz, *Death and the Right Hand* (Routledge, 2013), 48.

220 **"transitional period is indefinitely prolonged":** Robert Hertz, "A Contribution to a Study of the Collective Representation of Death," in *Saints, Heroes, Myths, and Rites: Classical Durkheimian Studies of Religion and Society,* eds. and trans. Alexander Riley, Sarah Daynes, and Cyril Isnart (Routledge, 2016), 144–45.

220 **Robert Hertz died in battle:** Robert Parkin, *The Dark Side of Humanity: The Work of Robert Hertz and Its Legacy* (Routledge, 2012).

221 **Rituals and ancestors are most often assigned:** Fenella Cannell, "Ghosts and Ancestors in the Modern West," in *A Companion to the Anthropology of Religion,* eds. Janice Boddy and Michael Lambek (John Wiley and Sons, 2013), 203.

221 **"rituals" and "ancestors" are terms that fit quite well:** Here I am drawing on literatures of secularism, death, and the body, for example, Talal Asad, "Thinking About the Secular Body, Pain, and Liberal Politics," in *Living and Dying in the Contemporary World: A Compendium,* eds. Veena Das and Clara Han (University of California Press, 2016); Talal Asad, "What Do Human Rights Do? An Anthropological Enquiry," *Theory & Event* 4, no. 4 (2000); Fenella Cannell, "English Ancestors: The Moral Possibilities of Popular Genealogy," *Journal of the Royal Anthropological Institute* 17, no. 3 (2011); Abou Farman, "Speculative Matter: Secular Bodies, Minds, and Persons," *Cultural Anthropology* 28, no. 4 (2013); Thomas W. Laqueur, "The Dead Body and Human Rights," in *The Body,* eds. Sean Sweeney and Ian Hodder (Cambridge University Press, 2002).

221 **"ancient beliefs about life after death":** Asad, "Thinking About the Secular Body," 662.

221 **"quasi-'religious' status":** Ibid., 663.

221 **"a measure of sanctity":** Ibid.

221 **"Respect the remains":** International Committee of the Red Cross, "The Missing and Their Families," January 16, 2003, 114; see also Adam Rosenblatt, "Chapter Three: Forensics of the Sacred," in *Digging for the Disappeared* (Stanford University Press, 2015).

221 **"a form of tribute":** Cannell, "English Ancestors," 472.

222 **"more than a technical process":** Verdery, *Political Lives of Dead Bodies,* 25.

222 **"meanings, feelings, the sacred":** Ibid.

222 **To neglect a full recognition of the sacred:** As Zoë Crossland observes: "In the theoretical literature the habitual emphasis on the detached 'mechanical objectivity' of Western scientific practice tends to act to foreclose the possibility of full recognition of the affective, religious, and sacred dimensions of forensic archaeological work." Crossland, "Archaeology of Contemporary Conflict," 296.

224 **"Through art":** Wystan Hugh Auden, *Secondary Worlds: Essays* (Random House, 1968), 141.

Epilogue

227 **"the country's best-known grave-digging detective":** Weil, "Clyde Snow."

227 **Fundación de Antropología Forense de Guatemala (FAFG):** For more information on the team's work, see Fafg.org.

227 **Equipo Argentino de Antropología Forense (EAAF):** To learn more about "Argentina Te Busca," known as "Help Us Find You" in English, the international campaign to identify children abducted during the dictatorship, see cancilleria.gob.ar/en/find-you. For more information on the team's work, see Eaaf.org.

228 **El Colectivo de Arqueología, Memoria e Identidad de Tucumán (CAMIT):** For more information on the team's work, see facebook .com/colectivotucuman/.

228 **In 2019, the team published a book:** Ataliva, Gerónimo, and Zurita, *Arqueología Forense y Procesos de Memorias.*

ABOUT THE TYPE

This book was set in Walbaum, a typeface designed
in 1810 by German punch cutter J. E. (Justus Erich)
Walbaum (1768–1839). Walbaum's type is more French
than German in appearance. Like Bodoni, it is a classical
typeface, yet its openness and slight irregularities give
it a human, romantic quality.